Nonpharmacological Therapies in the Management of Osteoarthritis

Editor

Yves Henrotin

Bone and cartilage Research Unit (BCRU)
Department of Motricity Sciences
University of Liège
Institute of Pathology, level +5
CHU Sart-Tilman
4000 Liège
Belgium

Associate Editors

Kim Bennell

Centre for Health, Exercise & Sports Medicine
Department of Physiotherapy, School of Health Sciences
University of Melbourne
Melbourne, VIC
Australia 3010

Francois Rannou

Professor of Medicine
Department of Rehabilitation, Institute of Rheumatology
Cochin Hospital, APHP
INSERM U747
University Paris Descartes
France

CONTENTS

FOREWORD

Considered as inevitable for decades, osteoarthritis (OA) is now regarded as a "real" disease rather than an unavoidable marker of aging, like white hairs or wrinkles. This changing face of the disease is mainly due to researchers and to patients: (i) researchers, because they have demonstrated that OA is not the simple consequence of passive wear and tear of the cartilage but the result of biological events, with many degradative and inflammatory processes involving multiple tissues, cell types, chemical and physical mediators, (ii) patients, because they rejuvenate year after year. Indeed, the age corresponding to the so-called "third age" has moved back each year because of an increased life expectancy (an increase of 2 months every year). How can we now consider a 65 year-old patient as an "old" person (although this was the case even 30 years ago)?! Thus, patients' behaviour is changing, fortunately more demanding, requiring more effective treatments for their symptoms, pain and function. They now need their knees, hips, and hands for their profession, travels, daily activities, sports, *etc*. Based on these patients' requests and given the exponential increase in incidence and prevalence of OA expected in the next years, societal costs will soon be abysmal. The three main risk factors for OA, aging, obesity and trauma, can only be amplified in the coming decade. The new lifestyles observed in industrialized countries lead to new leisure activities or sports that increase lower limb injuries, or instead multiply the time spent in front of screens of any kind that increases weight proportional to the sedentary time. It is therefore urgent to anticipate this situation by implementing methods of prevention possibly cheaper than potential targeted drugs to come for cure.

All national and international recommendations for the management of OA stress the importance of not neglecting the non-pharmacological treatments, not only for primary prevention, but also for secondary prevention. This book, consisting of chapters written by authors, who are international leaders in this field, highlights all the potential of non-pharmacological treatments for OA, from weight loss, to manual therapy, exercises, educational programs, crenobalneotherapy, acupuncture, insoles, footwear and dietetic supplements. The added-value of this book is undeniably the effort to keep an evidence-based approach in all the chapters although this is challenging: it is much more difficult to conduct studies methodologically perfect for these types of intervention than it is for drugs: placebo groups, blinding, randomisation are uneasy to define, as Dr. Marty's chapter points out.

I am grateful to Professor Yves Henrotin for the coordination of such a book that will be a *must* to serve as a source of information for health care professionals, primary care physicians, orthopaedists, rheumatologists, geriatricians, physiotherapists, and any other professionals committed to helping all these patients who have to cope with such a painful and disabling disease.

Pr Francis Berenbaum
OARSI Past-President

PREFACE

Osteoarthritis (OA) is one of the most prevalent and chronic diseases affecting the elderly. Its most prominent feature is the progressive destruction of articular cartilage which results in impaired joint motion, severe pain and ultimately disability. Its prevalence and its impact on daily life pose a significant public health problem. Today, a cure for OA remains elusive and the management of OA is largely palliative focusing on the alleviation of symptoms. Current recommendations for the management of OA include a combination of pharmacological and non-pharmacological treatments. The term "non-pharmacological" includes physical therapy and rehabilitation, "nutraceuticals" or food supplements and surgical treatments. This book focuses on physical therapies, rehabilitation and nutraceuticals, while surgical treatments are not discussed. All guidelines on OA management highlight the importance of weight loss and physical activity to improve the functional status of OA patients. Although they are not recommended, a number of other therapies are commonly used by physicians and physical therapists in their daily practice. These techniques are not recommended because their efficacy is not evidenced by strong clinical trials. This category includes electrotherapy, ultrasound, electromagnetic field, spa, hydrotherapy, *etc.* The clinical relevance of these techniques and the difficulties in conducting high quality trials assessing their efficacy are stated by authors. This book is really a guide of good clinical practice for all health care professionals in charge of patients with OA.

Pharmacological management of OA is dominated by analgesic, nonsteroidal anti-inflammatory drugs, and Symptomatic Slow Acting Drugs (SYSADOA) which constitute a new class of drugs characterised by a slow action on OA symptoms and a good tolerability. Some SYSADOA are nutraceuticals (*i.e.* glucosamine, chondroitin sulphate, avocado/soybean unsaponifiable) and are provided as dietary supplements or prescribed drugs according to the country and the product specifications. The absence of a clear definition and requirements for registration of nutraceuticals throws the scientists and practitioners into confusion. Often data coming from preclinical and clinical studies of prescribed drugs are extrapolated to over-the-counter products which differ considerably in source, formula, purity, rhythm and dose administrated. In fact, more than 30 nutraceutical products are marketed as potentially active in OA but few have demonstrated their efficacy and safety in human clinical trials. Clearly, in terms of regulations, there is a need to resolve the general confusion about whether nutraceuticals are food supplements or medicines. This book aims to review the available scientific evidence supporting the efficacy, and explaining the mechanism of action of nutraceuticals targeting OA. It also gives the recent advances in term of nutraceuticals nomenclature, classification and regulation.

Pr Yves Henrotin
Bone and cartilage Research Unit (BCRU)
Department of Motricity Sciences
University of Liège
Institute of Pathology, level +5
CHU Sart-Tilman
4000 Liège
Belgium

List of Contributors

Asplin Katie

Musculoskeletal Research Group, School of Veterinay Medecine and Science, Faculty of Medicine and Health sciences, University of Nottingham, Sutton Bonington Campus, Sutton Bonington, LE12 5RD, United Kingdom, s4086823@student.uq.edu.au

Beaudreuil Johann

Service de Rhumatologie, Hôpital Lariboisière, AP-HP, Université Paris 7, Paris, France, johann.beaudreuil@lrb.ap-hop-paris.fr

Bennell Kim

Centre for Health, Exercise & Sports Medicine, Department of Physiotherapy, School of Health Sciences, University of Melbourne, Melbourne, VIC, Australia, 3010, k.bennell@unimelb.edu.au

Berenbaum Francis

Pierre & Marie Curie University Paris VI, AP-HP Saint-Antoine Hospital, Paris, France, francis.berenbaum@sat.aphp.fr

Clutterbuck Abigail

Musculoskeletal Research Group, School of Veterinay Medecine and Science, Faculty of Medicine and Health sciences, University of Nottingham, Sutton Bonington Campus, Sutton Bonington, LE12 5RD, United Kingdom, Abigail.Clutterbuck@nottingham.ac.uk

Forestier Romain

Centre de recherche rhumatologique et thermale, 15, avenue Charles de Gaulle, 73100 Aix-les-Bains, France, romain.forestier@wanadoo.fr

Francon Alain

Centre de recherche rhumatologique et thermale, 15, avenue Charles de Gaulle, 73100 Aix-les-Bains, France, alain-francon@wanadoo.fr

Henrotin Yves

Bone and Cartilage Research Unit (BCRU), Department of Motricity Sciences, University of Liège, Institute of Pathology, level +5, CHU Sart-Tilman, 4000 Liège, Belgium, yhenrotin@ulg.ac.be, www.bcru.be

Hunt Michael

Department of Physical Therapy, University of British Columbia, Vancouver, Canada, michael.hunt@ubc.ca

Hinman Rana

Centre for Health, Exercise & Sports Medicine, Department of Physiotherapy, University of Melbourne, Melbourne, VIC, Australia 3010, ranash@unimelb.edu.au

Marty Marc

Rheumatology department, Henri Mondor Hospital, Creteil, France, marc.marty@free.fr

Mobasheri Ali

Musculoskeletal Research Group, School of Veterinay Medecine and Science, Faculty of Medicine and Health sciences, University of Nottingham, Sutton Bonington Campus, Sutton Bonington, LE12 5RD, United Kingdom, ali.mobasheri@nottingham.ac.uk

Perrot Serge

Service de Médecine Interne et Thérapeutique, INSERM U 987, Hotel Dieu Hospital, 1 Place du Parvis Notre Dame, 75004 Paris, France, Serge.perrot@htd.aphp.fr

Poiraudeau Serge

AP-HP, Service de Médecine Physique et Réadaptation, Hôpital Cochin, Université Paris Descartes, INSERM, Institut Fédératif de Recherche sur l'Handicap (IFR 25), 27 rue du faubourg Saint-Jacques, 75679 Paris Cedex 14, France, serge.poiraudeau@cch.aphp.fr

Rannou François

Université Paris Descartes, INSERM, Institut Fédératif de Recherche sur le Handicap (IFR 25), 27 rue du Faubourg Saint-Jacques, 75679 Paris Cedex 14, France, francois.rannou@cch.aphp.fr

Richette Pascal

Université Paris VII, UFR Médicale, Assistance Publique-Hôpitaux de Paris, Hôpital lariboisière, fédération de Rhumatologie, 75475 Paris Cedex 10, France, pascal.richette@lrb.aphp.fr

Sanchez Katherine

AP-HP, Service de Médecine Physique et Réadaptation, Hôpital Cochin, Université Paris Descartes, INSERM, Institut Fédératif de Recherche sur l'Handicap (IFR 25), 27 rue du faubourg Saint-Jacques, 75679 Paris Cedex 14, France, katherine.sanchez@cch.aphp.fr

Shakibaei Mehdi

Musculoskeletal Research Group, Institute of Anatomy, Ludwig-Maximilian - University of Munich, 80336 Munich, Germany, mehdi.shakibaei@med.uni-muenchen.de

Nonpharmacological Therapies in the Management of Osteoarthritis

CHAPTER 1

The Specific Challenges of Conducting High Quality Clinical Trials to Assess Conservative Non Pharmacological Treatments of Osteoarthritis

M. Marty*

Rheumatology Department, Henri Mondor Hospital, Creteil, France

Abstract: There is a need for health providers to disseminate the results of high quality trials to justify health care policy. Non pharmacological treatments (NPT) are recommended for the treatment of osteoarthritis (OA). NPT (including medical devices, technical interventions, participative interventions, and nutraceuticals) represent a wide range of treatments for OA. While the reference study design to evaluate the effects of NPT is the randomized controlled trial (RCT), other study designs are also appropriate. Specific methodological issues are associated with RCTs designed for the assessment of the efficacy of NPTs in OA. The key points of a high quality clinical trial protocol to assess the efficacy of NPT for the treatment of OA are presented and justified. The methodology proposed is mostly in line with the International Conference of Harmonization (ICH) guidelines, European Agency for the Evaluation of Medicinal Products (EMEA) recommendations and the recommended efficacy core sets for assessment of OA. Grading quality for RCT assessing NPT in OA is challenging. Four features represent specific challenges to conducting high quality RCTs assessing NPT in comparison with those assessing pharmacological treatment : 1) the potential influence of care providers on treatment (*e.g.* experience of a therapist for a physical therapy intervention), 2) the choice of comparator (waiting list, usual care, sham intervention, another NPT, or a pharmacological treatment), 3) the blinding of the intervention and 4) the methods of randomization and assignation of the intervention. Depending on the nature of the NPT, bias can be limited using adapted methodological issues but are often not fully avoided.

Keywords: Osteoarthritis, clinical trials, nonpharmacological treatments.

1. INTRODUCTION

Osteoarthritis (OA) is a frequent, chronic and non-life-threatening condition mainly characterized by pain, disability and impairment related to the affected joint (*e.g.* knee, hip, hand). These symptoms are recurrent, can worsen during painful episodes and diminish quality of life. The goals of symptom modifying treatments are to improve pain, function and quality of life. Health providers and scientists need results of high quality clinical trials to justify health care policy and recommendations. Decisions on the reimbursement of health care are then increasingly evidence based. Current recommended treatments of OA are divided into surgical, Pharmacological Treatments (PTs) and conservative non pharmacological treatments (NPTs) [1, 2, 3].

The Randomized Controlled Trial (RCT) is acknowledged as the most scientific rigorous study design for evaluating medical interventions. Grading quality for RCTs assessing NPT in OA is challenging. NPT evidence is systematically graded significantly lower methodologically than pharmacological therapy evidence for hip and knee OA [4, 5]. In general, the key points of a high quality RCT protocol designed to assess the efficacy of a NPT for the treatment of OA are the same as those assessing a pharmacological therapy. The quality of the RCT depends on the protocol, the conduct of the clinical trial, the analysis of the data and the reporting of results. Good Clinical Practice is an international ethical and scientific quality standard for designing, conducting, recording and reporting trials that involve the participation of human subjects [6]. A recent extension of the CONSORT (Consolidation Standards of Reporting Trials) for trials assessing non pharmacological treatments has been published [7].

---

*Address correspondence to M. Marty: Rheumatology Department, Henri Mondor Hospital 51, avenue du Maréchal-de-Lattre-de-Tassigny, 94000 Créteil, France; Tel: +33-1-49814703; E-mail: marc.marty@free.fr

Yves Henrotin, Kim Bennell and Francois Rannou (Eds)

Four features (because of source of bias in treatment effect) are very specific challenges to conducting high quality RCTs assessing NPT in comparison with those assessing pharmacological treatment: 1) the potential influence of care providers on NPT administration (*e.g.* experience of a therapist for a physical therapy intervention). OA is a heterogeneous condition and many NPT are considered as complex interventions including multimodal components. Intervention with NPT can be some times individualized to the patient based on clinical reasoning rather than standardized. To limit this source of bias, it is necessary to standardize the individualization of the NPT with written procedures and to give training to care providers, 2) the choice of the comparator (waiting list, usual care, sham intervention, another NPT, or a pharmacological treatment), 3) the blinding of the intervention and 4) the method of randomization and assignation of treatment.

This article describes the key clinical and methodological features of a RCT protocol designed to assess the efficacy of a NPT in OA. In the first part, the design and the methods are detailed, while those which do not raise specific issues and are commonly accepted and recommended for any RCT are briefly presented. In the second part, we address the specific issues of conducting the trial. Finally, the third part recalls the high quality data management rules and principles of statistical analysis. Finally guidelines for reporting trials are commented upon.

2. PROTOCOL FOR ASSESSING NON PHARMACOLOGICAL THERAPIES IN OA

The design and methods of clinical trials evaluating NPT should be in line with the International Conference of Harmonization (ICH) [6, 8], the Outcome Measures in Rheumatoid Arthritis Clinical Trials (OMERACT) III [9] and Consolidated Standards of Reporting Trials (CONSORT) Guidelines particularly its non-pharmacological extension [7, 10].

2.1. Background

The background section should explain the reasons justifying the conduct of a new clinical trial. A clinical trial evaluating the effect (efficacy and or safety) of a NPT on human volunteers can be performed because of lack of evidence on efficacy of this NPT, the need to evaluate efficacy in specific population, the particular need to compare a NPT to another treatment *etc.* The background section is usually built on previous clinical data on OA and on experience gained from previous research (including mechanisms which could explain efficacy) on the investigated NPT. According previous data the clinical trial should designed as confirmatory (to support efficacy with very precise hypotheses) or exploratory.

2.2. Design

Randomized controlled trials are widely recognized as being the best design for avoiding or minimizing bias in assessment of a treatment effect. The most common design of RCT is the parallel-group trial but other RCT designs such as cluster-randomized trials [11], patient-preference trials [12, 13], Zelen design trial [14-16], tracker trials [17, 18] and expertise-based RCTs [19] are also used (Table **1**).

The choice of the study design is influenced by the nature of the tested treatment [5]. For example, for the comparison of NPT (e.g: program of rehabilitation) versus an invasive technique (*e.g.* surgical technique), a patient-preference trials should be considered as an adapted design.

2.3. Objective

The primary objective of the study should be in accordance with the claimed and expected effect. This protocol section should include a brief description of the tested treatment and the comparator, the study population, the primary endpoint (*e.g.* change of pain between baseline visit and at 3 months visit) and the nature of the comparison (superiority or non inferiority between tested treatment and comparator).

2.4. Inclusion Criteria of Patients

The inclusion and exclusion criteria for patients with OA have been detailed in the literature. The selection of a patient (*e.g.* pain intensity, duration and severity of disease) should be in accordance with the assessed treatment. For example, the profile of patients included in a RCT to evaluate a surgical technique will be more severe than those of patients included in RCT assessing insoles. The symptoms should be of sufficient intensity at randomization to enable detection of a difference between the 2 groups. Selection of patients with mild intensity of pain would mean that the primary endpoint has little scope to change in a large number of patients, regardless of the placebo effect which is recognized to be substantial in OA [20]. Even among patients likely to experience change, it is necessary to select those with sufficiently severe OA to be able to distinguish between NPT and a comparator. If the 0 to 100 mm VAS (visual analogue scale) of pain intensity is used as the primary endpoint (see methodological considerations below), a VAS score of 40 mm or 50 mm at baseline could be considered as a sufficiently discriminative minimum severity cut off.

Table 1: Alternatives study design to conventional randomized clinical trial.

Study design	Principles	Main advantages	Main disadvantages
Cluster randomized trials	Randomization is performed on groups of patients. Examples: hospitals, department, geographic location.	To allow to evaluate a practice. To eliminate contamination of the intervention effects between patients within a cluster.	Larger sample (to assess cluster effect) Difficulty in blinding .
Patient preference trials	According preference of patients and willingness to be randomised, three groups of patients are considered : 1/ patients with no strong preferences and therefore consent to randomisation; 2/ patients with a preference who still consent to randomisation; 3/ patients who refuse randomisation and opt for their preferred treatment.	To study the influence of preference on outcome of treatment. To understand the generalization of results.	Larger sample Risk of major patient's influence predominant on endpoint.
Zelen design trial	Patients are blinded as to hypotheses.	To minimize the risk of refusing of consent of patients. Patients are not influenced by the fact to be not included in one group rather than the other. The control group is thus unaware that randomization has taken place.	Patients are not truly informed and it's a controversial method (ethical considerations).
Tracker trials	Used only for new and fast changing technologies. Protocol is flexible with an independent committee.	To avoid assessing new technology too late.	Complex design and complex statistic method. Need for an independent committee.

2.5. Treatment

NPT treatment should be described and standardized as precisely as possible to be reproducible by another team. Each component of NPT which may influence the estimated effect should be described. For rehabilitation programs, a quantitative (such as number of sessions, frequency of sessions, and duration of sessions) and qualitative description (such as nature of program, type of exercise) are required.

While it may be ideal to provide standardized treatment in a clinical trial, this is not necessarily reflective of clinical practice in which many NPTs are individualized taking into account patient presentation on clinical examination. Boutron *et al.* [4] reported that in 30% of 50 RCTs assessing NPT in hip and knee OA the treatment was individualized compared with only 3.3 % of the 60 trials assessing pharmacological treatment [4].

Contrary to pharmacological treatment, the treatment effects are likely to be influenced by the healthcare professional that performs the intervention. Given that the healthcare professional is an integral part of the intervention, some criteria of eligibility of the care provider should be addressed. These criteria should include the level of skill and experience of care provider. To avoid difference among care providers, training should be provided.

All dispositions should have taken to increase the adherence to the treatment (*e.g.* leaflet recalling to patients the treatment and the importance to be compliant, calls from nurses). Recording the adherence to the intervention is crucial to assess the accuracy of the results and the generalizability of results [13].

2.6. Comparator

The choice of the control group is a critical aspect of the design of any clinical trial. In a trial assessing NPT, it is often technically or/and ethically difficult to perform a placebo treatment. Comparators can be sham intervention, another NPT, a pharmacological treatment, a waiting list or a usual treatment. Sham intervention with no or limited "extra pharmacological" effects appears to be the best option, but this option is not always possible. If the control treatment is usual care, the protocol should indicate if care providers have to follow particular guidelines or are free to perform the care management as they usually do.

The choice of the comparator depends on the tested NPT:

- For participative interventions such as a physiotherapy program, educational program or spa therapy, either a control intervention of the same nature but with no rationale for efficacy or another participative intervention can be proposed.

- For devices, sham devices mimicking a test device can be proposed.

The comparator will have some consequence on the tested hypotheses. The lesser the efficacy of the control treatment, the greater the difference should be between the tested treatment and the comparator. Nevertheless, in any case, the comparator must be a choice acceptable for the patient in comparison with the tested intervention to facilitate patient adherence.

When the tested treatment and the comparator are different (*e.g.* rehabilitation program versus surgery) the trial can be an expertise-based RCT [19]. In that case, the provider performs only the intervention they can provide (*e.g.* surgeon).

So the comparator also influences the interpretation of the results and the conclusions that can be drawn. If a waiting list or no treatment is used as comparator, it is really difficult to conclude whether the observed difference between tested treatment and comparator can be linked with the direct effects of the treatment or with the effects of seeing a therapist.

2.7. Blinding

In a RCT assessing NPT, blinding is more difficult to obtain than in a RCT of pharmacological treatment [21, 22]. The lack of blinding may result in inaccuracy in the assessment of the treatment effect. It is therefore necessary to use some methodological techniques to reduce this bias [23].

Different blinding methods have to be considered: participants (patients), test treatment (or comparator), care providers, care providers of concomitant treatments and global care of patients, assessor of criteria, and the statistician. All these blinding methods should be described in the protocol. In most cases, the test treatment (or comparator if it is an NPT) providers cannot be blinded (*e.g.* a surgeon or a rehabilitation program) as a consequence of the nature of the treatment.

When blinding of the treatment is not possible, blinding of participants to the study hypothesis has been proposed by some authors. Partial information is given to participants (Zelen or Modified Zelen design) and they are randomized before the signature on the consent form [14, 16]. Nevertheless, this method is controversial [15]. In this method, patients are analysed in their assigned group even if they refuse to participate in the study.

When the tested treatment and comparator are different (*e.g.* rehabilitation program versus pharmacology treatment of tablets) a double dummy is possible. For example, a sham rehabilitation program is combined with tablets in the pharmacological treatment group and a placebo tablet is associated with the rehabilitation program in the rehabilitation program group.

In any case, the assessor of the main outcome criteria should be different and independent of the care providers and if possible should be blinded. But this precaution has a limited impact on reduction of bias because most of the recommended end points (pain, function, patient global assessment) in OA are patient outcome report such as Visual Analogue Scale (VAS) or Numerical Rating Scale (NRS).

2.8. Randomization

This point is very important, because of the difficulty in performing adequate blinding. Description of the generation of the list of randomization code should be described (such as stratification, and minimization). The method of allocating the patient to the tested intervention or comparator must protect against assigning patients to the intervention (test or comparator) with a risk of the predictability. One way to limit the risk of the predictability of treatment is the use of a centralized randomization system with an inter voice response system or an internet web response system.

To reduce the number of randomized patients who will not receive the assigned treatment, the time between randomization and the onset of intervention should be as short as possible. For example, in a trial comparing two methods of rehabilitation (one tested and one sham), randomization of patients should be performed just before the first day of the rehabilitation program rather than at the selection visit and performed by an investigator who is independent of the intervention.

2.9. Co-Treatment

As for any RCT, authorized and prohibited co-treatments should be described in the protocol to increase the causality of the results. Prohibited treatment must be stopped before the run-in period and prohibited throughout the study. Ideally, the protocol should also specify the authorized rescue medication and the procedure in case of non-authorized rescue medication intake. In a non inferiority trial this point is very important.

2.10. Duration of Treatment

OA is a chronic disease with acute episodes. Some treatments are designed to provide short-term alleviation, others are longer term. The duration (follow up) of the RCT should be adapted to the objective and the expected effect.

2.11. Prognostic Factors

It is important to specify baseline covariates and prognostic factors that are known to explain the efficacy primary endpoint, because adjusting for them increases statistical power. Also, subgroup analyses enable detection of differences in treatment effect across the covariates and prognostic factors levels. These factors can be stratified (in the randomization-the best) or adjusted at the time of statistical analysis or both. The prognostic factors should be adapted at the duration of the trial. A few possible factors in OA could be factors such as gender, disease severity, body mass index, knee alignment, *etc.*

2.12. Patient Withdrawals and Attrition of Sample

For different reasons patients can withdraw from the RCT after randomization and before or after the onset the intervention. To avoid incomplete outcome data related to withdrawal, assessment of efficacy and safety should be recorded at the time of withdrawal. Experienced investigators should avoid loss to follow up. Patients should be informed of the importance of the follow up and should be recalled by any way (mail, phone, e-mail, *etc.*) for their follow up visits. However, it is also important to note that all post randomization dropouts result in attrition bias. For example in a trial comparing a rehabilitation intervention to mini-invasive therapy (surgery), some patients may be excluded from analysis after randomization if the reason for withdrawal is independent of treatment and occurs before the intervention.

These patients should be described in the reporting of the trial. Loss to follow up can lead to bias in a RCT. Imbalance resulting from possible attrition should be recorded.

2.13. Endpoints

2.13.1. Primary Endpoint of Efficacy

A clinical endpoint is defined as a measure that allows decision of whether the null hypothesis of a clinical trial must be accepted or rejected. In a clinical trial assessing a NPT in OA, the choice of the primary endpoint should be founded on pain or function [18, 20]. Pain related to the target joint (hip or knee or hand) is recommended as the primary endpoint for symptom modifying treatment and functional disability should be considered as a co-primary endpoint. For pain Visual Analogue Scale (VAS) or Numerical Rating Scales (NRS, 0 -10) are self and validated methods. Functional disability should be assessed by validated tools such as WOMAC or Lequesne's index. Other parameters can then be used as secondary end points: patient global's assessment of disease activity, percentage of patients reaching Patient Acceptable Symptom State (PASS), percentage of patients achieving minimal improvement (Minimal clinically important improvement), Osteoarthritis Research Society International (OARSI) responder [24], onset of action, physician's global assessment of diease activity, total OA questionnaire, AUC pain intensity, quality of life, consumption of rescue medication [20]. As for any RCT, the null hypothesis should be fully described giving a precise definition of the primary endpoint.

2.13.2. Secondary Endpoints of Efficacy and Safety

Secondary efficacy end points, recording of adverse events and serious adverse should be also described.

2.14. Adherence

Assessing adherence to treatment (assignment and adherence) is essential to appraising the feasibility and the applicability of the intervention in clinical practice. However, defining parameters of the NPT intervention and checking adherence remains challenging. The better the NPT description, the easier the parameters of adherence are.

2.15. Sample Size

Sample size calculations are still inadequately reported in RCTs and are often erroneous and based on assumptions that are frequently inaccurate [25]. As in any RCT, the sample size estimate should be precisely described. The estimate is performed on the primary endpoint, with a type I error of 0.05 or less, a type II error of 0.20 or less, an estimated parameter of distribution of the main endpoints and an expected difference or non inferiority margin between the 2 groups. If an interim analysis is scheduled, justification, rules of decision and all requested statistical adjustment should be indicated. As Boutron *et al.* [7] highlight, if a cluster RCT is conducted, the sample size estimate should ideally be adjusted for the clustering effect.

2.16. Statistical Analysis

Statistical methods do not raise specific issues but they must be in accordance with the recommended statistical principles [8]. The main analysis of the primary end point should be precisely indicated: 1) the method of calculation of the primary endpoint (*e.g.* change of VAS of pain between baseline value and month 3 adjusted on baseline value), 2) the population considered for the main analysis (*e.g.*; full analysis set or per protocol), 3) the method to handle drop-outs and more generally missing data in the analysis, 4) the statistical test scheduled.

-   Usually three population sets are scheduled in the protocol:

    The safety population usually comprises all randomized patients who received at least a minimal exposure to the intervention. The Full Analysis Set (FAS) represents all randomized patients who have a baseline value and at least one post randomization value of the primary end point. In FAS, patients keep their assigned group even when they have not received the treatment. The per protocol population represents all patients of the FAS who have been exposed to the assigned intervention with a minimal level of adherence to intervention and who have a baseline value of the primary end point and one value of the end point (usually at the end of the study). In trials assessing NPTs the results can depend in part on the skill and training of the tested treatment (or comparator) care providers. Therefore, the center effect (care providers) should be tested. If a cluster RCT is conducted, cluster effect should be tested.

-   Another key methodological point is the management of drop-outs and missing data. Advances in the statistical theory of missing data over the last 20 years have shown that the most used approach for handling missing data, *i.e.* the Last Observation Carried Forward (LOCF) based method, systematically leads to a biased estimation of the treatment effect excepted the rather unrealistic approach assuming that the patient profile remains stable over time till the end of the trial [26]. In theory we know neither the size nor the direction of this bias. This analysis, which often leads to a conservative effect (which can easily be explained post hoc from configurations of observed missing data), has often been favored by the Regulators. However, such a method leading to a conservative effect that is biased to an unknown degree should not be recommended as the primary analysis. Currently, the simplest missingness mechanism which is not based on assumptions in addition to those of the observed data, and which is the subject of a consensus, is the 'Missing At Random' (MAR) mechanism [26]. This mechanism is valid if the missingness of the outcome assessed over time depends only on the previous observed data, but not on unobserved data. If this mechanism is valid, and if we have several VAS scores over time, it is shown that a mixed model for repeated measurements using maximum likelihood estimation provides an unbiased treatment effect at the selected time endpoint (*e.g.* three months). We therefore recommend assessing the primary outcome endpoint at intermediate time points so as to conduct the primary analysis in the mixed model for repeated measurements. The LOCF method could then be presented as a sensitivity analysis, since the Regulatory Authorities often require its use, while stressing its inherent dangers of interpretation. As the validity of the MAR mechanism cannot be checked in practice, other sensitivity analyses of the primary analysis could be done, assuming more sophisticated mechanisms of generating missing data (*e.g.*, missing not at random mechanisms). These accept that the missingness of the primary outcome assessed over time can also depend on unobserved data, so as to "frame" the results of the primary analysis more rigorously than that based on the LOCF method.

-   In any case, given possible bias of the main analysis of the primary end point, sensitivity analysis of the primary end point should be conducted. Sensitivity analysis is performed on the primary end points with another method than used for the primary analysis: e.g; using sample (per protocol population, completer), another statistical tests, different techniques for considering missing data, adjusted analysis considering different factors as prognosis factors, centers. These analyses provide information on the robustness of the results with the primary analysis of the primary end point.

3. CONDUCTING THE CLINICAL TRIAL

Good Clinical Practice (GCP) [6] is an international ethical scientific quality standard for designing, conducting, recording and reporting clinical trials involving humans. Clinical trials should be conducted in accordance with principles of ICH GCP. Compliance with these principles provides assurance that the rights, safety and well being of trial subjects are protected and that the clinical trial data are credible. GCP should also contribute to avoiding incomplete outcome data.

Responsibilities of Independent Ethics Committee (IEC), investigators, and sponsor are well defined (GCP). Essential documents requested for the conduct of a clinical trial are also described.

4. DATA MANAGEMENT AND ANALYSIS OF DATA

Recording of data on Case Report Forms (CRF) or in e-CRF by investigators should be monitored according to GCP. Careful data management (checking all inconsistencies) will help ensure a valid data base is obtained. Good Clinical Data Management Practice (GCDMP) is the current industry standard for clinical data management that consist of best business practice and acceptable regulatory standards. The Society of Clinical Data Management (SCDM) has created a comprehensive document that provides guidance on accepted practices of Clinical Data Management (CDM) that are not totally covered by FDA guidelines and regulations. This document is entitled Good Clinical Data Management Practices (GCDMP) and version 4.0 was most recently published in May 2007 (http://www.scdm.org/gcdmp/).

To avoid any discussion after analysis a precise data management plan should be written. Before breaking the code of randomization by the statistician, a careful blind review of data should be conducted to determine the minor and major deviation to the protocol allowing determination of safety population, FAS (full analysis set) considered as the intention-to-treat population and per protocol population [6].

For the analysis, main analysis of the primary end points should be conducted as it was scheduled in the protocol and in the statistical analysis plan. This plan should contain all information necessary to conduct the statistical analysis of the RCT.

5. REPORTING

Reporting of a clinical trial depends on the protocol, the data management and the statistical analysis. A note for guidance on the structure and content of the clinical study report is available [27]. Simply ethics considerations, investigators, administrative structure implicated in the study, background and investigational plan should be recalled. All changes in the study management or in the statistical plan should be described.

Publication in a peer review journal with a high impact factor is the best way to disseminate the data. Negative and positive studies should be published. Editors are responsible for ensuring the quality of their journals and that what is reported is ethical, accurate and relevant to their readership. Peer review must involve assessment by external reviewers. A report in a journal of a RCT should be transparent for the reader, explain why the RCT has been undertaken and how it was conducted and analyzed. Any factor which is not precisely described and can include a bias in treatment effect limits the interpretation of the results. The CONSORT (Consolidation Standards of Reporting Trials) has established a checklist of 22 items and flow diagram for reporting RCT and this checklist has been revised in 2001 [22]. The 22 items concerns title and abstract (1 item) introduction (1 item), methods (10 items), results (7 items) and discussion (3 items). A recent extension of the CONSORT (Consolidation Standards of Reporting Trials) for trials assessing NPT has been published [7] and highlights the specific topics to report RCT assessing a NPT. Most of these specific topics have been developed in this article. Furthermore Clinical Trial Registration is required by the International Committee of Medical Journal Editors and it is recommended to register a RCT prior to commencing recruitment.

CONCLUDING REMARKS

RCTs are scientific investigations that examine and evaluate the safety and efficacy of new drugs or therapeutic procedures using human subjects. The results that these studies generate are considered as the most valued data in the era of evidence based medicine. Unbiased RCTs are requested to avoid any over- or under-estimate of the treatment effect.

Developing high quality trials RCT of NPT in patients with OA is achievable and should be pursued wherever possible. Conventional randomized trials are widely recognized as the most reliable method to evaluate PT and should be conducted as often as possible. Unfortunately, the treatment effect estimates generated in RCT assessing NPT are rarely free of errors (bias, confounding factors, and random error).

Depending of the nature of NPT, questions remain about the use of conventional RCT to evaluate NPT. The challenges are defining control interventions, blinding and assignation to group. Some methods are available to minimize bias (*e.g.* selection of patients, study management, blinding, and analysis) but sometimes it is not enough in a conventional RCT. Under circumstances in which major bias of a conventional RCT are expected, designs such, cluster-randomized trials [11], patient-preference trials [12, 13]), Zelen design trial [14-16], tracker trials [17, 18] and expertise-based RCTs [19] could, however, be used as alternative [5]. In any case a balance must be struck between the risk of providing a biased treatment effect and the difficulty of conducting trials with a very low risk of bias. A better understanding of the risks of bias may result in an improved design, conducting and reporting of trials, with a closer estimate of the true effectiveness of an intervention as a result.

REFERENCES

[1]   Zhang W, Doherty M, Arden N, *et al.* EULAR evidence based recommendations for the management of hip osteoarthritis: report of a task force of the EULAR Standing Committee for International Clinical Studies Including Therapeutics (ESCISIT). Ann Rheum Dis 2005; 64: 669-81.

[2]   Zhang W, Moskowitz EW, Nuki G *et al.* OARSI recommendations for the management of hip and knee osteoarthritis, part II : OARSI evidence-based, expert consensus guidelines. Osteoarthritis Cartilage 2008; 16: 137-162.

[3]   Osteoarthritis. The care and management of osteoarthritis in adult (2009). Nice guideline 59. available on www.nice.org.uk/GC059.

[4]   Boutron I, Tubach F, Gireaudeau B, Ravaud P. Methodological differences in clinical trials evaluating non pharmacological and pharmacological treatments of hip and knee osteoarthritis. JAMA 2003; 290:1062-70.

[5]   Ravaud Ph, Boutron I. Primer: assessing the efficacy and safety of non pharmacologic treatments for rheumatic diseases. Nat Rev Rheumatol 2006; 2: 313-319.

[6]   Note for guidance on good clinical practice. CPMP/ICH/135/95. July 2002.

[7]   Boutron I, Poher D, Altman DG, Schultz KF, Ravaud Ph. Extending the CONSORT statement to randomized trials of non pharmacological treatment : explanation and elaboration. Ann Intern Med 2008; 148: 295-309.

[8]   Note for guidance on Statistical principles for clinical trials. CPMP/ICH/363/96. September 1998.

[9]   Bellamy N, Kirwan J, *et al.* Recommendations for a core set of outcome measures for future phase III clinical trials in knee, hip, and hand osteoarthritis.Consensus development at OMERACT III. J Rheumatol 1997; 24: 799-802.

[10]   Moher D, Schulz KF, Altman DG. The CONSORT statement: revised recommendations for improving the quality of reports of parallel group randomized trials. Lancet 2001; 357:1191-1194.

[11]   Mallick U, Bakhai A, Wang D, Flather M. Cluster randomized trials. In Wang D, Bakhai A, Eds. Clinical Trials. London. Remedica 2007; pp 141 -151.

[12]   Preference Collaborative Review Group. Patients'preferences within randomised trials : systematic review and patients level meta-analysis. BMJ 2008; 337: a1864.

[13]   Torgerson D, Sibbald B, General practice. Understanding controlled trials: What is a patient preference trial? BMJ 1998; 316: 360.

[14]   Zelen M. A new design for randomized clinical trials. N Engl J Med 1979; 300: 1242-5.

[15]   Homer CS. Using the Zelen design in randomized controlled trials: debates and controversies. J Adv Nurs 2002; 38: 200-207.

[16]   Campbell R, Peters T, Grant C, Quilty B, Dieppe P. Adapting the randomised consent (Zelen) design for trials of behavioural interventions for chronic disease: feasibility study. J Health Sev Res Policy 2005; 10: 220-225.

[17]   Schroeder TV. Evidence-based medicine in rapidly changing technologies. Scand J Surg 2008; 97: 100-104.

[18]   Lilford RJ, Braunholtz DA, Greenhalgh R, Edwards SJ. Trials and fast changing technologies: the case for tracker studies. BMJ 2000; 320: 43-46.

[19]   Devereaux PJ, Bhandar M, Clarke M *et al.* Need for expertise based randomised controlled trials. BMJ 2005; 330: 1-5.

[20]   Guideline on clinical investigation of medicinal products used in the treatment of osteoarthritis. CPMP/EWP/794/97 Rev 1 August 2010.

[21]   Gluud LL. Bias in clinical intervention research. Am J Epidemiol. 2006; 163:493-501.

[22]   Jüni P, Altman DG, Egger M. Systematic review in health care. Assessing the quality of reports of controoled clinical trials. BMJ 2001; 323:42-6.

[23] Boutron I, Guittet L, Estellat C, Moher D, Hrobjartsson A, Ravaud P. Reporting methods of blinding in randomized trials assessing non pharmacological treatments. PLoS Med 2007; 4: e61. doi: 101371/journal.pmed.00400061.

[24] Pham T, Van der Heijde D, Altman RD, Anderson JJ, Bellamy J, Hochberg M. OMERACT-OARSI initiative: Osteoarthritis Research Society International set of responder criteria for osteoarthritis clinical trials revisited. Osteoarthritis Cartilage 2004; 12: 389-99.

[25] Charles P, Giraudeau B, Dechartes A, Baron B Ravaud P. Reporting of sample size calculation in randomised. Controlled trials: review. BMJ 2009; 338: b1732.

[26] Molenberghs G, Thijs H, Jansen I, Beunckens C. Analysing incomplete longitudinal clinical trial data. Biostatistics 2004; 5: 445-464.

[27] Note for guidance on structure and content of clinical study reports. CPMP/ICH/137/95) July 1996.

CHAPTER 2

Nonpharmacological Approaches in Management of Hip and Knee Osteoarthritis-Related Pain

S. Perrot[*]

Hôtel Dieu, Service de Médecine Interne, Université Paris 5 Descartes, Paris, France

Abstract: Non-pharmacological approaches are highly recommended for osteoarthritis (OA) treatment to reduce pain and improve function and quality of life. Based on international recommendations for the management of OA, we summarize herein the non-pharmacological treatments that may exhibit some analgesic effects in knee and hip OA. Studies on analgesic non-pharmacological approaches in OA include exercise, patient education, orthoses, acupuncture, physical agents and balneotherapy. Even though many of the published studies have methodological issues, it can be concluded that some of these approaches demonstrate analgesic effects with fewer side effects compared with pharmacological treatments. More evidence is available for knee OA than for hip OA for most of the nonpharmacological treatments. In all cases, these approaches should be individualised to each patient and can be combined together as well as combined with pharmacological management.

Keywords: Pain, osteoarthritis, exercise, alternative treatment, education.

1. INTRODUCTION

Osteoarthritis (OA) is a chronic joint condition, characterized by pain, disability, and impairment. The main treatment goals include pain relief, improved function, slowed disease progression and enhanced quality of life. Guidelines on the management of OA recommend both pharmacological and non-pharmacological approaches [1] and many patients also use complementary and alternative medicines. An increasing number of systematic reviews are available regarding non-pharmacological and nonsurgical interventions. While studies generally score lower in terms of methodological quality than those involving pharmacological agents [2], non-pharmacological treatments represent interesting approaches to pain management. Assessment of non-pharmacological treatments must take into consideration methodological issues and the fact that pain in OA is complex. In this chapter we will summarize the non-pharmacological approaches for pain in hip and knee OA.

2. EXERCISE

Exercise is one of the most important non-pharmacological treatments for symptomatic hip and knee OA. It increases muscle strength and facilitates weight loss. Analysis of the literature demonstrates that effects are more marked on function than on pain, and that effects appear to be more significant for knee OA than for hip OA.

Effect sizes in exercise interventions are small to moderate for both pain and functional improvements and are similar to those observed for improvement in pain with Non-Steroidal Anti-Inflammatory Drugs (NSAIDs) [3-5]. However, in contrast to NSAIDs, exercise interventions are safe and can improve pain and function through a direct effect on muscle strength and function. Both aerobic and strengthening exercises seem to be equally effective with regard to pain and function in patients with OA. Fransen *et al.* have [6] demonstrated that group exercise sessions are as effective as individual exercise therapy (standardized response mean 0.42 for individual exercise versus 0.65 for group therapy). In their systematic review, based on 5 high quality and 6 low-quality studies, Pisters *et al.* [7] demonstrated that the positive post-treatment effects of exercise therapy on pain and physical function in patients with OA of the hip

*Address correspondence to S. Perrot: Service de Médecine Interne et Thérapeutique, INSERM U 987, Hotel Dieu Hospital, 1 Place du Parvis Notre Dame, 75004 Paris, France; Tel: +33 1 42 34 84 49; Fax : +33 1 42 34 85 88; E-mail: Serge.perrot@htd.aphp.fr

Yves Henrotin, Kim Bennell and Francois Rannou (Eds)

and/or knee are not sustained in the long term. Long-term effectiveness was only found for patient global assessment of effectiveness. However, additional booster sessions after the treatment period positively influenced long-term maintenance of beneficial post-treatment effects on pain and physical function.

Among exercise modalities, aquatic approaches are of interest in hip and knee OA. In their meta-analysis of aquatic exercises in hip and knee OA, Bartels *et al.* [8] demonstrated a lack of high-quality studies with a total of six trials (800 participants) included. When combining hip and knee OA, there was a small-to-moderate effect on function (SMD 0.26, 95% confidence interval (CI) 0.11 to 0.42) and a small-to-moderate effect on quality of life (SMD 0.32, 95% CI 0.03 to 0.61). A minor effect of a 3% absolute reduction (0.6 fewer points on a 0 to 20 scale) and 6.6% relative reduction from baseline was found for pain. When studying hip OA alone, no evidence of effect on pain, function or quality of life was observed in the single trial. When studying knee OA alone, one trial comparing aquatic exercise with land-based exercise demonstrated a large effect on pain (SMD 0.86, 95%CI 0.25 to 1.47; 22% relative percent improvement), but no evidence of effect on stiffness or walking ability. Only two studies reported adverse effects, that is, the interventions did not increase self-reported pain or symptom scores. In a trial involving 786 participants aged 45 years or over, Thomas *et al.* [9] demonstrated that at a 24 month follow-up, highly significant reductions in knee pain were apparent for the pooled exercise groups compared with the non-exercise group, but with similar improvements at 6, 12 and 18 months. The reduction in pain was greater the closer patients adhered to the exercise plan.

Whereas most of the data are related to knee OA, the lack of evidence on the effectiveness of exercise for OA joints other than the knee is of concern [10]. Two high-quality reviews reported on the effects of exercise on hip OA [11, 12]. Fransen *et al.* [13] concluded that no optimal exercise type or dosage could be identified due to little available scientific evidence. Roddy *et al.* [14] concluded that there is some evidence that strengthening exercise may be beneficial in reducing pain in people with hip OA, but that there is not enough evidence to make conclusions on its effect on disability. There also is not enough evidence to make conclusions about the effect of aerobic exercise on pain, disability, or health status.

3. SELF-MANAGEMENT STRATEGIES AND EDUCATION

As in many chronic conditions, several self-management programs have been proposed in painful musculoskeletal conditions. In rheumatology, educational programs have been developed since the eighties [15] but recently programs have been also developed for OA.

These educational programs aim to:

-   Coordinate multidisciplinary approaches: symptomatic treatments, local injections, psycho-social management, diet, orthoses, adapted to patients' objectives and issues;

-   Manage pharmacological treatment side-effects: putative analgesic and anti-inflammatory side-effects, especially in elderly patients [16];

-   Optimize surgical strategies, especially joint replacement.

One of the key self-management programs in OA is the Arthritis Self Management Programs (ASMP) [17]. It is derived from the Stanford Self Management Program and has been developed by Kate Lorig, a famous nurse, involved in patient education and self-management approaches in rheumatology [18]. This program has been tested in several studies in the US and UK that have confirmed the usefulness and efficacy of this approach on pain, quality of life and disability. Results are globally good, depending on the methodology and the studied population, and demonstrate a positive impact on pain, function [17], and even on healthcare cost-effectiveness [18]. MacCarthy *et al.* [19] have also demonstrated a sustained efficacy (24 months) on pain and function of a home-based educational program, added to rehabilitation exercises. Ravaud *et al.* [20] demonstrated that standardized visits with specific tasks and messages at each visit have a superior impact on pain, function, weight loss and quality of life, compared to usual visits to rheumatologists.

As in other non-pharmacological approaches, studies on self-management in OA have methodological issues such as no double-blinding, randomization, or inclusion of a control group. Globally, Warsi *et al.* [21], in their review on self-management in chronic conditions have demonstrated some benefit in OA: these programs included coping strategies training, pain management, exercises, cognitive approaches, and identification of problems. In most cases, patient education is not provided alone but combined with rehabilitation [22].

4. ORTHOTIC DEVICES

The third EULAR recommendation is dedicated to the non-pharmacological approach in the treatment of knee OA [23] and orthotic devices are recommended mainly on the basis of expert opinion, not evidence.

One randomized clinical trial, comparing one group with a knee sleeve, one group with a valgus brace and a control group without a knee sleeve or a brace, has been described [24]. This study showed a significant improvement in pain and function for the two intervention groups. In addition, valgus brace treatment is more effective than a simple knee sleeve. A Cochrane review on orthoses and braces [25] concluded that there is limited evidence that (a) a brace has additional beneficial effects (WOMAC, MACTAR, function tests) for knee OA compared with medical treatment alone, (b) a sleeve has additional beneficial effects (WOMAC, function tests) for knee OA compared with medical treatment alone, (c) a brace is more effective (WOMAC, function tests) than a neoprene sleeve (d) a laterally wedged insole can decrease NSAIDs intake, (e) patient compliance is better with a laterally wedged insole compared with a neutral insole, (f) a strapped insole has more adverse effects than a lateral wedge insole. These findings are for knee OA since no recommendations on orthoses in hip OA have been published.

4.1. Wedges

The use of a lateral wedge insole is believed to lower knee medial compartment load and reduce lateral tensile forces by enhancing *valgus* correction of the calcaneus, whether or not *varus* deformity at the knee is lessened. Rodrigues *et al.* [26] have demonstrated that the use of medial-wedge insoles was highly effective in reducing pain at rest and on movement and promoted a functional improvement of *valgus* knee OA.

4.2. Braces

Braces may be used to transfer load to the normal, or at least less diseased, compartment of the knee in order to reduce pain from the narrowed joint compartment. Toda *et al.* [27] studied the effectiveness of a simple hinged brace and a *valgus* corrective brace in 12 patients with OA of the medial compartment. Significant improvements in pain, function and loading and propulsive forces were seen with the *valgus* brace, however the simple brace only showed improvements in loading forces. Both braces improved confidence and function during gait. It may be concluded that the use of knee bracing appears to be clinically effective, however the long-term effectiveness and with that the indication and limitations have to be established [27].

4.3. Knee Taping

Knee taping is a simple, inexpensive method believed to relieve pain by improving alignment of the patella-femoral joint and/or unloading inflamed soft tissue, but there is little evidence to justify its use. Hinman *et al.* [28] performed a randomized single blind controlled trial (87 participants with OA) with three intervention arms (therapeutic tape, control tape, and no tape) of three weeks' duration and a three week follow up. A significant effect on pain was observed at three weeks ($p<0.001$), with 73% (21/29) of the therapeutic tape group reporting improvement compared with 49% (14/29) of the control tape group and 10% (3/29) of the no tape group. Benefits of therapeutic tape were maintained three weeks after stopping treatment. These results indicate that therapeutic knee taping is an effective treatment for the management of pain and disability in patients with knee OA; however further studies evaluating long term effects of knee taping are required.

5. ACUPUNCTURE

Although acupuncture may reduce pain and improve both physical function and related quality of life, and is widely used by patients, little evidence of its effectiveness is observed in knee OA [29], with no evidence for hip OA.

5.1. Acupuncture in Knee OA

Witt *et al.* [30] performed a randomized controlled trial to investigate acupuncture in addition to routine care, compared with routine care alone, in the treatment of 3633 patients with chronic pain due to OA of the knee or hip. At 3 months, the WOMAC score had improved significantly in the acupuncture group compared with the control group. Similarly, quality of life improvements were significantly greater in the acupuncture group (p<0.001). Treatment success was maintained through 6 months.

These findings were confirmed by another study from Witt *et al.* [30] in knee OA. This study investigated the efficacy of acupuncture compared with minimal acupuncture and with no acupuncture: after 8 weeks of acupuncture treatment, pain and joint function (WOMAC scores) were improved significantly compared with minimal acupuncture or no acupuncture.

A multicentre, randomized trial investigated the benefit of adding acupuncture (true and non-penetrating acupuncture) to a course of advice and exercise delivered by physiotherapists for pain reduction in patients with knee OA. Compared with advice and exercise alone there were small, statistically significant, improvements in pain intensity and unpleasantness at two and six weeks for true acupuncture and at all follow-up points for non-penetrating acupuncture. The small additional benefits from acupuncture were unlikely to be clinically significant, mostly short lived, and could not be attributed to specific acupuncture needling effects; therefore further research is needed to investigate the possible mechanisms of acupuncture, particularly the role of expectancy effects [31].

Vas *et al.* [32] demonstrated that acupuncture added to NSAIDs in the treatment of knee OA, was more effective than NSAIDs alone. Acupuncture treatment provided to the intervention group (true acupuncture plus diclofenac) significantly reduced pain, improved physical capability and psychological functioning compared with the control group (placebo acupuncture plus diclofenac).

5.2. Acupuncture in Hip OA

One high-quality systematic review [33] assessed the effect of acupuncture in individuals with hip OA. The conclusions were based on three primary studies. On the basis of the meta-analysis, there were no statistically significant results, and thus there was no evidence that acupuncture is beneficial for reducing hip OA pain. Mean pain reduction was 14.43 (on a 0–100 Visual Analog Scale [VAS]) for the intervention group and 15.31 for the sham treatment group (mean difference of - 0.03, 95% confidence interval [CI] = - 0.52 – 0.45).

6. PHYSICAL AGENTS

Bjordal *et al.* [34] have published a meta-analysis on efficacy of physical agents and indicated that within the 4 first weeks, manual acupuncture, static magnets and ultrasound therapies did not offer statistically significant short-term pain relief over placebo.

6.1. Pulsed Ultrasound

Pulsed ultrasound has been recommended for acute pain and inflammation. A recent revised Cochrane review concluded that in contrast to the previous review, ultrasound may be beneficial for patients with OA of the knee [35]. Because of the low quality of the evidence, the authors were uncertain about the magnitude of the effects on pain and function, but nevertheless they recommend the use of pulsed ultrasound in knee OA. A recent study confirmed a slight but significant effect on pain related to knee OA [36].

6.2. Pulsed Electromagnetic Field Therapy (PEMF)

PEMF used for delayed-union fractures has also been suggested as an alternative treatment for OA. Physical stress on bone leads to the appearance of piezoelectric potentials that may act as the transduction signals that promote bone formation. It is thought that similar mechanism exists in cartilage that stimulates chondrocytes to increase proteoglycan synthesis. However a six week double-blind placebo-controlled randomized trial found that there was no significant difference between active magnet pulse and sham treatment groups in pain reduction, WOMAC score or EuroQol score [37]. A recent study [38] failed to demonstrate significant analgesic effects of pulsed electromagnetic fields in knee OA.

Harlow *et al.* [39] performed a randomized controlled trial of magnetic bracelets in 194 people with hip or knee OA aged 45-80 years. Participants were divided into groups wearing a standard strength static bipolar magnetic bracelet, a weak magnetic bracelet, or a non-magnetic (dummy) bracelet for 12 weeks. Mean pain scores were reduced more in the standard magnet group than in the dummy group (mean difference 1.3 points, 95% CI:0.05 - 2.55). Thus it was concluded that pain from OA of the hip and knee decreases in patients wearing magnetic bracelets.

6.3. Electrical Stimulation Therapy

Electrical stimulation therapy was found to have a small to moderate effect on knee OA pain. In a placebo-controlled trial of Pulsed Electrical Stimulation (PES), Garland *et al.* [40] reported a better response for the active device than for the placebo device on pain, physical function, physician global assessment and duration of joint stiffness in the morning ($p<0.05$). No statistically significant difference was observed for range of knee joint motion, joint tenderness, joint swelling, knee circumference and 50 feet walking time.

In a prospective cohort study of 288 (95 men, 193 women) patients using a PES device for 16 to more than 600 days (mean: 889 hours) Far *et al.* [41] demonstrated an improvement in all efficacy variables ($p<0.001$). Furthermore, there was a dose-response relationship between effect size and hours of usage: improvement in 59% of patients who used it less than 750 hours compared with 73% of those who used it more than 750 hours. An economic analysis of a sub-group of patients showed that 45.3% reduced NSAIDs use by 50.0% or more. Thus a highly optimized PES device successfully attenuated knee OA symptoms in patients who had failed non-surgical therapy.

6.4. TENS (Transcutaneous Electrical Nerve Stimulation)

In their 2009 Cochrane review, Osiri *et al.* [42] concluded from seven trials that TENS is effective in controlling pain compared with placebo. Heterogeneity of the included studies was observed which might be due to the different study designs and outcomes used. More well designed studies with a standardized protocol and adequate numbers of participants are needed to conclusively determine the effectiveness of TENS in the treatment of OA of the knee.

6.5. Low Level Laser Therapy

In their 2007 Cochrane review that included five trials Brosseau *et al.* [43] showed a statistically significant difference favoring laser treatment when compared to placebo for at least one outcome measure. Three trials did not report beneficial effects. The varying results of these trials may be due to the method of laser application and/or other features of laser application. There is clearly a need to investigate the effects of different dosages of low level laser therapy in future randomized, controlled clinical trials in OA.

7. HYDROTHERAPY AND SPA

Several studies suggest an overall beneficial effect of spa therapy in chronic musculoskeletal diseases and this treatment has been particularly appreciated by elderly people for many years. Several literature reviews have been performed on hydrotherapy and spa therapy. A Cochrane review [44] concluded that there was slight evidence of an analgesic effect of mineral baths compared to no treatment. No clear effect was found with other balneological treatment, in part due to low methodological quality of studies. More recently,

Harzy *et al.* [45] concluded that all interventions used in these studies found improvements in pain and functional capacity that were sustained until week 24. No serious adverse events were reported to be associated with thermal mineral waters treatment. A recent and important study [46] has been published to determine whether spa therapy, home exercises and usual medical treatment provides any benefit over exercises and usual treatment, in the management of knee OA. At 6 months, 50.8% of the spa group patients demonstrated clinically meaningful changes, compared to 36.4% controls (p=0.005).

Additional randomized controlled trials with similar intervention comparisons and outcome measures are required to confirm these results and to assess the biological effect of thermal mineral water in patients with knee OA.

8. THERMOTHERAPY

In painful OA, especially in knee OA, patients frequently use hot or cold packs. A Cochrane review performed in 2003 by Brosseau *et al.* [47] concluded that ice massage had a statistically beneficial effect on range of motion, function and knee strength compared to control. Cold packs decreased swelling but did not significantly affect pain. Hot packs had no beneficial effect on edema compared with placebo or cold application. More well designed studies with a standardized protocol and adequate numbers of participants are needed to evaluate the effect of thermotherapy in the treatment of knee OA.

CONCLUDING REMARKS

In summary, non-pharmacological approaches in OA may be effective in relieving pain, with more evidence available for knee OA than for hip OA. However, analgesic effects related to non-pharmacological approaches are weak and non-sustained, except for spa therapy where long lasting effects up to 24 weeks may be demonstrated. Most of the non-pharmacological treatments appear safer than pharmacological treatments [48]. Furthermore, treatments can be combined together and also combined with pharmacological approaches. Unfortunately many of the studies investigating non-pharmacological treatments have low methodological quality scores. In the future, additional studies seeking responders related to specific techniques as well as optimal combinations of pharmacological and non-pharmacological treatment should be conducted.

REFERENCES

[1]   Zhang W, Doherty M, Arden N, *et al.* Eular recommendations for hip osteoarthritis: report of a task force of the EULAR Standing Committee for International Clinical Studies Including Therapeutics (ESCISIT). Ann Rheum Dis 2005; 64: 669-681.

[2]   Boutron I, Tubach F, Giraudeau B, Ravaud P. Methodological differences in clinical trials evaluating nonpharmacological treatments of hip and knee osteoarthritis. JAMA 2003; 290: 1062-1070.

[3]   DeAngelo N, Gordin V. Treatment of patients with arthritis-related Pain. JAOA 2004; 104(11): 2-5.

[4]   Bischoff HA, Roos EM. Effectiveness and safety of strengthening, aerobic, and coordination exercises for patients with osteoarthritis. Curr Opin in Rheumatol 2003; 15: 141-44.

[5]   Hunter DJ, Felson DT. Osteoarthritis. BMJ 2006; 332: 639-42.

[6]   Fransen M, Crosbie J, Edmonds J. Physical therapy is effective for patients with osteoarthritis of the knee: a randomized controlled trial. J Rheumatol 2001; 28: 156-64.

[7]   Pisters MF, Veenhof C, van Meeteren NL, *et al.* Long-term effectiveness of exercise therapy in patients with osteoarthritis of the hip or knee: a systematic review. Arthritis Rheum 2007; 57: 1245-53.

[8]   Bartels EM, Lund H, Hagen KB, Dagfinrud H, Christensen R, Danneskiold-Samsøe B. Aquatic exercise for the treatment of knee and hip osteoarthritis. Cochrane Database Syst Rev 2007; 4:CD005523.

[9]   Thomas KS, Muir KR, Doherty M, Jones AC, O'Reilly SC, Bassey EJ. Home based exercise programme for the knee pain and knee osteoarthritis: randomized, controlled trial. BMJ 2002; 325: 752-56.

[10]   Dieppe P, Brandt KD. What is important in treating osteoarthritis? Whom should we treat and how should we treat them? Rheum Dis Clin N Am 2003; 29: 687-716.

[11]   Fransen M, McConnell S, Bell M. Exercise for osteoarthritis of the hip or knee. Cochrane Database Syst Rev 2003;(3):CD004286.

[12]   Roddy E, Zhang W, Doherty M, *et al.* Evidence-based recommendations for the role of exercise in the management of osteoarthritis of the hip or knee: the MOVE consensus. Rheumatology (Oxford). 2005;44:67-73.

[13]   Mullen PD, Laville EA, Biddle AK, Lorig K: Efficacy of psychoeducational interviews on pain, depression, and disability in people with arthritis: MetaAnalysis. J Rheum 1987; 14: 33-39.

[14]   Superio-Cabuslay E, Ward MM, Lorig KR: Patient education interventions in osteoarthritis and rheumatoid arthritis: a meta-analytic comparison with non steroidal anti-inflammatory drug treatment. Arthritis Care Res 1996, 9:292-301.

[15]   Lorig K, Mazonson P, Holman H: Evidence suggesting that health education for self-management in patients with chronic arthritis has sustained health benefits while reducing health care costs. Arthritis Rheum 1993, 36:493-496.

[16]   Lorig K. Partnership between expert patients and physicians. The Lancet 2002, 359:814-815.

[17]   Coleman S, Briffa K, Conroy H, Prince R, Carroll G, McQuade J. Short and medium-term effects of an education self-management program for individuals with osteoarthritis of the knee, designed and delivered by health professionals: a quality assurance study. BMC musculoskelet dis 2008; 9: 117.

[18]   Offman JJ, Badamgarav E, Henning JM, *et al.* Does disease management improve clinical and economic outcomes in patients with chronic diseases? A systematic review. Am J Med 2004; 117: 182-192.

[19]   McCarthy CJ, Mills PM, Pullen R, *et al.* Supplementation of a home-based exercise programme with a class-based programme for people with osteoarthritis of the knees: a randomised controlled trial and health economic analysis. Health Technol Assess 2004; 8 (46).

[20]   Ravaud P, Flipo RM, Boutron I, et.al. ARTIST (osteoarthritis intervention standardized) study of standardised consultation versus usual care for patients with osteoarthritis of the knee in primary care in France: pragmatic randomised controlled trial. BMJ 2009; 23: 338 (b421).

[21]   Warsi A, Wang PS, LaValley MP, Avorn J, Solomon DH. Self-management education programs in chronic disease. A systematic review and methodological critique of the literature. Arch Intern Med 2004; 164:1641-1649.

[22]   Yip YB, Sit JW, Wong DY, Chong SY, Chung LH. A 1-year follow-up of an experimental study of a self-management arthritis programme with an added exercise component of clients with osteoarthritis of the knee. Psychol Health Med 2008; 13: 402-14.

[23]   Jordan KM, Arden NK, Doherty M *et al.* and Standing Committee for International Clinical Studies Including Therapeutic Trials ESCISIT. EULAR recommendations 2003: an evidence based approach to the management of knee osteoarthritis: Report of a Task Force of the Standing Committee for International Clinical Studies Including Therapeutic Trials (ESCISIT). Ann Rheum Dis 2003; 62: 1145-55.

[24]   Kirkley A, Webster-Bogaert S, Litchfield R *et al.* The effect of bracing on varus gonarthrosis, J Bone Joint Surg 1999; 81: 539-548.

[25]   Brouwer RW, Jakma TS, Verhagen AP, Verhaar JA, Bierma-Zeinstra SM. Braces and orthoses for treating osteoarthritis of the knee. Cochrane Database Syst Rev 2005; 25: CD004020.

[26]   Rodrigues PT, Ferreira AF, Pereira RM, Bonfá E, Borba EF, Fuller R. Effectiveness of medial-wedge insole treatment for valgus knee osteoarthritis. Arthritis Rheum 2008; 59(5): 603-8.

[27]   Toda Y, Tsukimura N. A 2-year follow-up of a study to compare the efficacy of lateral wedged insoles with subtalar strapping and an in-shoe lateral wedged insoles in patients with varus deformity osteoarthritis of the knee. Osteoarthritis Cartilage 2005; 14: 231-37.

[28]   Hinman RS, Crossley KM, McConell J, Bennell KL. Efficacy of knee tape in the management of osteoarthritis of the knee: blinded randomised controlled trial. BMJ 2003; 327: 135-40.

[29]   Witt CM, Jena S, Brinkhaus B, Liecker B, Wegscheider K, Willich SN. Acupuncture in patients with osteoarthritis of the knee or hip: a randomized, controlled trial with an additional nonrandomized arm. Arthritis Rheum 2006; 54(11): 3375-7.

[30]   Witt C, Brinkhaus B, Jena S, *et al.* Acupuncture in patients with osteoarthritis of the knee: a randomised trial. Lancet 2005; 366 (9480): 136-43.

[31]   Foster NE, Thomas E, Barlas P *et al.* Acupuncture as an adjunct to exercise based physiotherapy for osteoarthritis of the knee: randomised controlled trial. BMJ 2007; 335: 436-47.

[32]   Vas J, Mendez C, Perea-Milla E *et al.* Acupuncture as a complementary therapy to the pharmacological treatment of osteoarthritis of the knee: randomized controlled trial. BMJ 2004; 329: 1216-21.

[33]   Kwon YD, Pittler MH, Ernst E. Acupuncture for peripheral joint osteoarthritis. Rheumatology (Oxford) 2006; 27:1-7.

[34] Bjordal JM, Johnson MI, Lopes-Martins RA, Bogen B, Chow R, Ljunggren AE. Short-term efficacy of physical interventions in osteoarthritic knee pain. A systematic review and meta-analysis of randomised placebo-controlled trials. BMC musculoskelet dis [serial online] 2007 June.

[35] Rutjes AW, Nüesch E, Sterchi R, Jüni P. Therapeutic ultrasound for osteoarthritis of the knee or hip. Cochrane Database Syst Rev 2010; 1:CD003132.

[36] Ozgönenel L, Aytekin E, Durmuşoglu G. A double-blind trial of clinical effects of therapeutic ultrasound in knee osteoarthritis. Ultrasound Med Biol 2009; 35(1): 44-9.

[37] Pipitone N, Scott DL. Magnetic pulse treatment for knee osteoarthritis: a randomized, double-blind, placebo-controlled study. Curr Med Res Opin 2001; 17: 190-6.

[38] Ay S, Evcik D. The effects of pulsed electromagnetic fields in the treatment of knee osteoarthritis: a randomized, placebo-controlled trial. Rheumatol Int 2009; 29(6):663-6.

[39] Harlow T, Greaves C, White A, Brown L, Hart A, Ernst E. Randomised controlled trial of magnetic bracelets for relieving pain in osteoarthritis of the hip and knee. BMJ 2004; 329: 1450-4.

[40] Garland D, Holt P, Harrington JT, Caldwell J, Zizic T, Cholewczynski J. A 3-month, randomized, double-blind, placebo controlled study to evaluate the safety and efficacy of a highly optimized, capacitively coupled, pulsed electric stimulator in patients with osteoarthritis of the knee. Osteoarthritis Cartilage 2007; 15(6): 630-7.

[41] Farr J, Mont MA, Garland D, Caldwell JR, Zizic TM. Pulsed electrical stimulation in patients with osteoarthritis of the knee: follow up in 288 patients who had failed non-operative therapy. Surg Technol Int 2006; 15: 227-33.

[42] Osiri M, Welch V, Brosseau L *et al.* Transcutaneous electrical nerve stimulation for knee osteoarthritis. Cochrane Database Syst Rev Rev 2009; (4):CD002823.

[43] Brosseau L, Robinson V, Wells G *et al.* WITHDRAWN: Low level laser therapy (Classes III) for treating osteoarthritis. Cochrane Database Syst Rev 2007; 1:CD002046.

[44] Verhagen AP, Bierma-Zeinstra SM, Boers M *et al.* Balneotherapy for osteoarthritis. Cochrane Database Syst Rev. 2007; 4:CD006864. Review. PubMed PMID: 17943920.

[45] Harzy T, Ghani N, Akasbi N, Bono W, Nejjari C. Short- and long-term therapeutic effects of thermal mineral waters in knee osteoarthritis: a systematic review of randomized controlled trials. Clin Rheumatol 2009; 28: 501-7.

[46] Forestier R, Desfour H, Tessier JM. Spa therapy in the treatment of knee osteoarthritis: a large randomised multicentre trial. Ann Rheum Dis 2010; 69: 660-5.

[47] Brosseau L, Yonge KA, Robinson V. Thermotherapy for treatment of osteoarthritis. Cochrane Database Syst Rev 2003; (4): CD004522.

[48] Sakalauskiene G, Jauniskiene D. The use of nonpharmacological approaches in management of osteoarthritis. Medicinos 2010; 16(2):166-74.

CHAPTER 3

Non-Pharmacological Therapies for the Management of Osteoarthritis in Guidelines: Discrepancies and Translating Evidence in Practices

Y. Henrotin[*]

Bone and Cartilage Research Unit, University of Liège, Institute of Pathology, Level +5, CHU Sart-Tilman, 4000 Liege, Belgium

Abstract: Osteoarthritis (OA) refers to a syndrome of joint pain accompanied by functional limitation and reduced quality of life. The treatment of OA syndrome is dominated by pharmacological treatments, including analgesics and non-steroidal anti-inflammatory drugs that relieve symptoms but fail to modify disease progression. However, according to the most popular guidelines for good management of OA, the optimal treatment requires a combination of non-pharmacological and pharmacological treatments. The chapter gives a critical analysis of the most popular recommendations for the non-pharmacological management of knee, hip and hand OA. This chapter provides useful guidance and support for health care professionals making treatment decisions. It also describes the barriers to implement OA guidelines in clinical practice.

Keywords: Osteoarthritis, recommendations, knee, hip.

1. INTRODUCTION

Osteoarthritis (OA) is one of the most common chronic musculoskeletal conditions worldwide, with a growing socio-economic impact. Commonly, the hip and knee are mostly affected by OA, therefore most of the existing recommendations are focused on these joints. In 2007, the Osteoarthritis Research Society International (OARSI) published a critical appraisal of the existing treatment guidelines for hip and knee OA [1]. Twenty-three guidelines were identified in MEDLINE, EMBASE, AMED, CINAHL and the Science citation index database. Six guidelines were predominantly based on opinion, five primarily based on evidence and 12 based on both. OARSI then used the (Appraisal of Guidelines Research and Evaluation) AGREE instrument to evaluate the quality of all existing guidelines for scope and purpose, stakeholder participation, methodological rigour and overall quality, clarity, applicability and editorial independence. Overall quality was better in evidence-based than in opinion-based guidelines, and significantly better still in the hybrid guidelines that combined research evidence with expert opinion. Whilst the majority of the guidelines did not separate hip and knee, eight were specific for the knee, but only one for the hip. Thirteen guidelines had been developed for specific care settings (five for primary care, three for rheumatology, three for physiotherapy and two for orthopaedics), but ten did not specify target users. Fifty-one treatment modalities were addressed in the 23 guidelines. Twenty of these modalities were recommended by all of the guidelines in which they were addressed. These included non pharmacological modalities of therapy aerobic exercise (21/21 guidelines), strengthening exercise (21/21), education (15/15), self-management (8/8), water-based exercise (8/8), regular telephone contact (2/2) and cane/stick (11/11). By contrast, weight loss, Transcutaneous Electrical Nerve Stimulation (TENS) and patellar tape were recommended in 13/14, 8/10 and 12/13 of the guidelines respectively, where these modalities were considered. Finally, heat/ice, acupuncture and massage were recommended in 7/10, 5/8 and 1/2 guidelines respectively, while ultrasound and laser were recommended in less than 50% of the guidelines where these modalities were addressed. In general, non-pharmacological therapies had a numerically smaller effect size (ES) for pain (ES=0.25, 95% CI 0.16, 0.34) than pharmacological therapies (ES = 0.39, 95% CI 0.31, 0.47). Taken individually, the effect size for pain or function of non-pharmacological modalities ranged between 0.06 to 1.13. The lower pain or function ES was recorded for self-management, education and ultrasound modalities whereas the

*Address correspondence to Y. Henrotin:** Bone and Cartilage Research Unit, University of Liège, CHU Sart-Tilman, 4000 Liège, Belgium; Tel: +32 4 3662516; Fax : +32 4 3664734; E-mail: yhenrotin@ulg.ac.be.

Yves Henrotin, Kim Bennell and Francois Rannou (Eds)

higher ES was calculated for heat/ice. Interestingly, the cost/QALY ratio was $10,483 USD for water-based exercise, $22,297 for acupuncture but $61,915 for non steroidal anti-inflammatory drugs (NSAIDs) + proton pump inhibitor (PPI) and $60,367 for COX-2 selective NSAIDs.

The first recommendations for the diagnosis, investigation and management of hip and knee OA were issued by the Royal College of Physicians in 1993. Subsequently, the American College of Rheumatology (ACR) developed guidelines for knee and hip OA [2, 3] and the European League Against Rheumatism (EULAR) [4-6] developed guidelines on knee OA then hip OA and finally hand OA. Recently, international recommendations on knee and hip OA were proposed by OARSI [7], and holistic recommendations on OA were published by the National Institute for Health and Clinical Excellence (NICE) [8]. Finally, in 2010, the ACR published updated recommendations for hand, hip and knee OA [9]. In general, these recommendations included both non-pharmacological and pharmacological modalities.

This chapter is a critical analysis of the recommendations published on the non-pharmacological, non-surgical management of OA. We have extracted recommendations for non-pharmacological modalities from ACR (Table **1**), EULAR (Table **2**), OARSI (Table **3**) and NICE (Table **4**) guidelines and compared them. The selection of guidelines discussed in this paper is arbitrary and was based mainly on the following criteria: editorial independence, based on both evidence and opinion, quality, applicability and accessibility.

In this chapter nutraceuticals are excluded from the non-pharmacological therapies. This point has been already addressed in several systematic review and meta-analysis [10, 11]. This chapter also compares the methods used to produce these guidelines and the results. Finally, it investigates whether these guidelines are being implemented into clinical practice.

Table 1: List of the ACR recommendations for non-pharmacological therapies in the management of knee and hip OA.

Knee OA
Strong recommendation
1. Cardiovascular and resistance land-based exercise.
2. Aquatic exercise.
3. Weight loss (for persons who are overweight)
Weak recommendation (suggest)
4. Participation in self-management programs
5. Manual therapy in combination with supervised exercise
6. Psychological interventions
7. Medially directed patellar taping
8. Medially wedged insoles for persons with lateral compartment OA
9. Laterally wedged subtalar strapped insoles for persons with medial compartment OA.
10. Thermal agents
11. Walking aids
12. Traditional Chinese acupuncture*
13. Transcutaneous electrical stimulation*
No recommendation
14. Balance exercises, either alone or in combination with strengthening exercises
15. Tai Chi
16. Laterally wedged insoles
17. Manual therapy alone
18. Braces
19. Laterally directed patellar taping
Hip OA
Strong recommendation
20. Cardiovascular and resistance land-based exercise

21. Aquatic exercise
22. Weight loss (for persons who are overweight)

Weak recommendation (suggest)

23. Participation in self-management programs
24. Manual therapy in combination with supervised-exercise
25. Psychological interventions
26. Thermal agents
27. Walking aids

No recommendation

28. Balance exercises, either alone or in combination with strengthening exercises
29. Tai chi
30. Manual therapy alone

Hand OA

Weak recommendation (suggest)

31. Evaluation of ability to perform activities of daily living
32. Instruction in joint protection techniques
33. Provision of assistive devices, as needed
34. Instruction in use of thermal modalities
35. Splints for patients with trapezometacarpal joint OA

Table 2: List of the EULAR recommendations for non-pharmacological therapies in the management of knee, hip and hand OA.

Knee OA

1. Non-pharmacological treatment of knee OA should include regular education, exercise, appliances (sticks, insoles, knee bracing) and weight reduction.

Hip OA

1. Non-pharmacological treatment of hip OA should include regular education, exercise, appliances (stick, insoles) and weight reduction if obese or overweight.

Hand OA

1. Education concerning joint protection (how to avoid adverse mechanical factors) together with an exercise regimen (involving both range of motion and strengthening exercises) is recommended for all patients with hand OA.
2. Local application of heat (for example, paraffin wax, hot pack), especially before exercise, and ultrasound are beneficial treatments.
3. Splint for thumb base OA and orthoses to prevent/correct lateral angulations and flexion deformity are recommended.

2. METHODS FOR DEVELOPING RECOMMENDATIONS ON NON-PHARMACOLOGICAL MODALITIES

Well-defined methods exist for developing recommendations. The modern guidelines (*e.g.* OARSI, ACR 2010, NICE) use the Grades of Recommendation Assessment, Development and Evaluation (GRADE) approach [12]. Briefly, the GRADE approach to the development of evidence-based recommendations involves the following steps: 1) establishing the process; 2) preparing systematic reviews of the best available evidence for all modalities; 3) preparing evidence profiles for each modality for pre-specified clinically important outcome(s); 4) grading the quality of the evidence for each intervention by each pre-specified outcome; 5) balancing the benefits and risks of each intervention and 6) formulating the strength of each recommendation. In general (EULAR, OARSI, ACR), the estimated outcomes include Effect-Size (ES), number of patients needed to treat, relative risks or odds ratios and cost per-quality adjusted life year gained, the applicability of the evidence to the population of interest, practicability of delivery and economic considerations. The results of the review are then examined by a panel of experts, who ideally should come from several different countries and medical and allied health disciplines. A consensus is then obtained on proposals of recommendations elaborated on the basis of the literature review and in one case on clinical scenarios elaborated by experts (ACR 2010) [9]. In the majority of the guidelines, consensus recommendations were produced following a Delphi exercise and the Strength of Recommendation (SOR) for propositions relating to each modality was even determined using a visual analog scale (*e.g.* OARSI).

3. WHAT DO THE MAIN RECOMMENDATIONS SAY?

3.1. General Recommendations (Applicable to all Joints)

3.1.1. Combination of Pharmacological and Non-Pharmacological Modalities

Optimal management of OA requires a combination of pharmacological and non- pharmacological treatment modalities (EULAR 2000, 2003, 2005, 2007 [4, 6, 13, 14]; ACR 1995 [3], OARSI 2008[7]).

3.1.2. Patient-Centered Care

Treatment of OA should be individualized according to the localization of OA, specific (*i.e.* adverse mechanical factor, physical activity and obesity for hip and knee OA) and general risk factors (age, sex), type of OA (nodal, erosive, traumatic), presence of inflammation, severity of structural change, level of pain, disability, and restriction of quality of life, co-morbidity, and co-medication, and the wishes, preferences and expectations of the patient (EULAR 2000, 2007 [6, 13]; NICE 2008 [8]).

People with OA should have the opportunity to make informed decisions about their care and treatment, in partnership with their healthcare professionals. If the patient agrees, families and carers should have the opportunity to be involved in decisions about treatment and care (NICE 2008 [8]).

3.1.3. Information, Education and Self-Management

All patients with OA should be given information access and education, and where appropriate, education provided for the patient's family, friends or other caregivers about the disease and its therapy (ACR 1995, 2000 [2, 3, 15]; OARSI 2008 [7], NICE 2008 [8]). Practitioners should always explain to the patient the nature of their condition, its prognosis, the requirement of any investigations and what they involve, and determine with the patient the rationale and practicalities of their individualized management plan (EULAR 2000 [13], NICE 2008 [8]). The importance of changes in lifestyle, exercise, pacing of activities, weight reduction, and other measures to unload the damaged joint(s) should also be addressed (OARSI 2008 [7]). The initial focus should be on self-help and patient driven treatments rather than on passive therapies delivered by health professionals. Subsequently emphasis should be placed on encouraging adherence to the regimen of non-pharmacological therapy (OARSI 2008 [7]).

Information sharing should be an ongoing, integral part of the management plan rather than a single event at time of presentation (NICE 2008 [8]). Evidence-based written information tailored to the patient's needs should be used to support communication between healthcare professionals and patients (NICE 2008 [8]).

Education techniques shown to be effective include individualized education package, regular telephone calls, patient coping skills and spouse-assisted coping skills training (EULAR 2000, 2003 [13, 14]). Patients with OA should be encouraged to participate in a self-management program (ACR 1995, 2000 [2, 3]; NICE 2008 [8]).

3.1.4. To Refer the Patient at a Physical Therapist

The physical therapist assesses muscle strength, joint stability, and mobility; recommends the use of modalities such as heat (especially useful just prior to exercises) (ACR 2000 [15]); instructs patients in an exercise program to maintain or improve joint range of motion and periarticular muscle strength; performs manual therapy techniques; and provides assistive devices, such as canes, crutches, or walkers, to improve ambulation (ACR 2000 [15]; OARSI 2008 [7], NICE 2008[8]).

3.1.5. Assessment

A healthcare professional should assess the effect of OA on an individual's function, quality of life, occupation, mood, relationships and leisure activities (NICE 2008 [8]).

3.1.6. Regular Telephone Contact

Personalized social support through telephone contact to discuss such issues as joint pain, medications and treatment compliance, drug toxicities, date of next scheduled visit and barriers to keeping clinic appointments showed moderate-to-large degrees of improvement in pain and functional status without a significant increase in costs (ACR 2000 [15]).

3.1.7. Exercises

Exercises should be a core treatment for people with OA, irrespective of age, co-morbidity, pain severity or disability (NICE 2008 [8]). Patients with OA should be encouraged to undertake, and to continue to undertake, a regimen of exercises involving range of motion, joint-specific strength and general aerobic conditioning (EULAR 2000, 2007 [6, 13], ACR 2000 [15], OARSI 2008 [7], NICE 2008 [8]).

Table 3: List of the OARSI recommendations for non-pharmacological therapies in the management of hip and knee OA.

1. All patients with hip and knee OA should be given information access and education about the objectives of treatment and the importance of changes in lifestyle, exercise, pacing of activities, weight reduction, and other measures to unload the damaged joints. The initial focus should be on self-help and patient driven treatments rather than on passives therapies delivered by health professionals. Subsequently emphasis should be placed on encouraging adherence to regimen of non-pharmacological therapy.

2. The clinical status of patients with hip and knee OA can be improved if patients are contacted regularly by phone.

3. Patients with symptomatic hip and knee OA may benefit from referral to a physical therapist for evaluation and instruction in appropriate exercises to reduce pain and improve functional capacity. This evaluation may result in provision of assistive devices such as canes and walkers, as appropriate.

4. Patients with hip and knee OA should be encouraged to undertake, and continue to undertake, regular aerobic, muscle strengthening and range of motion exercises. For patients with symptomatic hip OA, exercises in water can be effective.

5. Patients with hip and knee OA, who are overweight, should be encouraged to lose weight and maintain their weight at a lower level.

6. Walking aids can reduce pain in patients with hip and knee OA. Patients should be given instruction in the optimal use of a cane or crutch in the contra-lateral hand. Frame and wheeled walkers are ore often preferable for those with bilateral disease.

7. In patients with knee OA and mild/moderate varus or valgus instability, a knee brace can reduce pain, improve stability and diminish the risk of falling.

8. Every patient with hip or knee OA should receive advice concerning appropriate footwear. In patients with knee OA insoles can reduce pain and improve ambulation. Lateral wedged insoles can be symptomatic benefit for some patients with medial tibio-femoral compartment OA.

9. Some thermal modalities may be effective for relieving symptoms in hip and knee OA.

10. TENS can help with short term control in some patients with hip or knee OA.

11. Acupuncture may be of symptomatic benefit in patient with knee OA.

3.1.8. Thermotherapy

Some thermal modalities (heat and cold therapy) may be effective for relieving symptoms in OA (OARSI 2008 [7]). The use of local heat or cold therapy should be considered as an adjunct to core treatment (exercises) (NICE 2008 [8]).

3.1.9. Self-Management Intervention

Self-management can be defined as any activity that individuals do to promote health, prevent disease and enhance self-efficacy. Self-management principles empower the patient to use their own knowledge and skills to access appropriate resources and build on their own experiences of managing conditions. Individualized self management strategies should be agreed between healthcare professionals and the persons with OA. Positive behavioral changes such as exercise, weight loss, use of suitable footwear and pacing should be appropriately targeted (NICE 2008 [8]).

Table 4: List of the NICE recommendations for non-pharmacological therapies in the management of OA.

1. Health care professionals should assess the effect of OA on the individual's function, quality of life, occupation, mood, relationships and leisure activities.
2. People with symptomatic OA should have periodic review tailored to their individual needs.
3. Health care professionals should formulate a management plan in partnership with the person with OA.
4. Co-morbidities that compound the effect of OA should be taken into consideration in the management plan.
5. Healthcare professionals should offer people with clinically symptomatic OA advice on the following core treatments: access to appropriate information, activity and exercise, interventions to effect weight loss if overweight or obese.
6. The risks and benefits of treatment options, taking into account co-morbidities, should be communicated to the patient in ways that can be understood.
7. Healthcare professionals should offer accurate verbal and written information to all people with osteoarthritis to enhance understanding of the condition and its management, and to counter misconceptions, such as that it inevitably progresses and cannot be treated. Information sharing should be ongoing, integral part of the management plan rather than a single event at time of presentation.
8. Individualised self-management strategies should be agreed between healthcare professionals and the person with OA. Positive behavioral changes such as exercise, weight loss, use of suitable footwear and pacing should be appropriately targeted.
9. Self-management programmes, either individually or in groups, should emphasise the recommended core treatments for people with OA, especially exercise.
10. The use of local heat or cold should be considered as an adjunct to core treatment.
11. Exercise should be a core treatment for people with OA, irrespective of age, comobidity, pain severity or disability. Exercise should include: local muscle strengthening, general aerobic fitness.
12. Manipulation and stretching should be considered as an adjunct to core treatment, particularly OA of the hip.
13. Intervention to achieve weight loss should be a core treatment for people who are obese or overweight.
14. Healthcare professionals should consider the use of transcutaneous electrical nerve stimulation (TENS) as an adjunct to core treatment.
15. Electro-acupuncture should not be used to treat people with OA.
16. Healthcare professionals should offer advice on appropriate footwear (including shock absorbing properties) as part of core treatment for people with lower limb OA.
17. People with OA who have biomechanical joint pain or instability should be considered for assessment for bracing/joint supports/insoles as an adjunct to their core treatment.
18. Assistive devices (for example, walking sticks and tap turners) should be considered as adjuncts to core treatment for people with OA who have specific problems with activities of daily living. Healthcare professionals may need to seek expert device in this context (for example from occupational therapists or disability equipment assessment centres).

3.1.10. Transcutaneous Electrical Nerve Stimulation (TENS)

Transcutaneous Electrical Nerve Stimulation (TENS) can help with short-term pain relief in some patient with OA (OARSI 2008 [7]) and should be considered as an adjunct of care treatment for pain relief (NICE 2008 [8]).

3.1.11. Acupuncture/Electro-Acupuncture

According to the NICE guidelines, electro-acupuncture should not be used to treat people with OA (NICE 2008 [8]). In contrast, OARSI recommends acupuncture to relieve pain in patient with knee OA (OARSI 2008 [7]).

3.1.12. Aids and Device

People with OA who have biomechanical joint pain or instability should be considered for assessment for bracing /joint supports/insoles as an adjunct to their core treatment (NICE 2008 [8]).

3.2. Recommendations Specific for Knee and Hip Osteoarthritis

3.2.1. To Lose Weight

To lose weight and to maintain their weight at a lower level is recommended for overweight patients with hip or knee OA (ACR, 1995, 2000 [2, 15], OARSI 2008 [7]). Interventions to achieve weight loss should be a core treatment for people who are obese or overweight (NICE 2008 [8], EULAR, 1995 [4]).

3.2.2. Aerobic Activities

A program of aerobic activity, supervised fitness walking program, cardiovascular and resistance land-based or aquatic exercises should be suggested to all patients with hip or knee OA to improve functional status and reduce pain (ACR 2000, 2010 [9, 15], EULAR 2000 [13]). The ACR 2010 expressed no preference for aquatic exercises as opposed to land-based exercises based on efficacy and safety; the decision should be individualized and based on patient preferences and ability to perform exercises.

3.2.3. Manual Therapy

Manual therapy in combination with supervised exercises, but not manual therapy alone is weakly recommended in knee and hip OA management (ACR 2010 [9]).

3.2.4. Walking Aids

Walking aids are recommended to reduce pain. Patients should be given instruction in the optimal use of a cane or a crutch in the contra-lateral hand. Frames or wheeled walkers are often preferable for those with bilateral disease (ACR 2000 [15]; OARSI 2008 [7], NICE 2008[8]).

3.2.5. Lifestyle and Assistive Devices

The patient may be taught principles of joint protection and energy conservation. For example, selected patients might be advised to live on one floor of their homes and to avoid stair climbing, when possible. Assistive devices, including raised toilet seats, dressing sticks for putting on socks and hose, and wall bars for getting in and out of a bathtub can be provided (NICE 2008 [8]).

3.2.6. Footwear

Every patient with hip or knee OA should receive advice concerning appropriate footwear (including shock absorbing properties and heel height) (OARSI 2008 [7]). This modality should be a part of core treatment for people with lower limb OA (NICE 2008 [8]).

3.3. Recommendations Specific for Knee OA

3.3.1. Quadriceps Strengthening

Quadriceps weakness is common among patients with knee OA. It is a manifestation of disuse atrophy, which develops because of unloading of painful extremity, but may also be present in persons with radiographic changes of OA who have no history of knee pain, and in whom lower extremity muscle mass is increased, rather than decreased, suggesting an arthrogenous origin of muscle weakness. Quadriceps weakness may be a risk factor for the development of knee OA, presumably by decreasing stability of the knee joint and reducing the shock absorbing capacity of the muscle (ACR 2000 [15]).

Exercises, especially those directed toward increasing strength of quadriceps (either isometric or isotonic) are strongly recommended to improve knee pain and function (ACR 2000 [15], EULAR 2000 [13], OARSI 2008[7]). If the patient cannot participate in an organized exercise program, the primary care physician should ensure that all he/she is instructed in quadriceps strengthening exercises (ACR 1995 [3]).

3.3.2. To lose Weight

The overweight patients with OA of the knee, especially if they are being considered as candidates for total knee replacement should be encouraged to participate in a comprehensive weight management program including dietary counseling and aerobic exercises (ACR 1995[3]). Specific dietary and other unproven therapies are not recommended in the management of patients with knee OA.

3.3.3. Insoles

Patients may benefit from shoe inserts to correct abnormal biomechanics due to angular deformities of the knee (ACR 1995 [3]). Lateral wedge insoles can be of symptomatic benefit for some patients with medial tibio-femoral compartment OA (OARSI 2008 [7]). The wearing of shock-absorbing shoes with insoles is believed to be of benefit (ACR 1995 [3]). The 2010 ACR recommendations give some additional precision [9]. Medially wedged insoles were weakly recommended for persons with lateral compartment OA and laterally wedged subtalar strapped insoles were recommended for persons with medial compartment. In contrast, no recommendation has been formulated for laterally wedged insoles without subtalar strapping.

3.3.4. Braces

The use of light-weight knee braces may also be helpful in patients with tibio-femoral disease, especially if complicated by lateral instability, for reducing pain, improving function and diminishing the risks of falling (ACR 1995 [3]; EULAR 2003[14], OARSI 2008[7]). No recommendations have been formulated for braces in ACR 2010.

3.3.5. Taping

In patients with symptomatic patello-femoral compartment OA, medial taping of the patella is recommended (ACR 2005, ACR 2010).

3.4. Recommendations Specific for hip OA.

3.4.1. Exercises

The goals of an exercise program are to preserve at least 30° of flexion and full extension of the hip, and to strengthen the hip abductors and extensors (ACR 1995[2]).

3.4.2. Cane

Proper use of a cane (in hand contralateral to the affected hip) reduces the loading forces on the joint and is associated with decreased pain and improved function (ACR 1995 [2]).

3.4.3. Shoes and Insoles

Patients may benefit from using shoe orthoses to correct abnormal biomechanics due to leg length inequality, as well as wearing shoes with viscoelastic insoles to decrease shock of impact loading (ACR 1995[2]).

3.4.4. Sexual Counseling

For patients with OA of the hip who have pain and/or difficulties with sexual activties, sexual counseling can be provided (ACR 1995[2]).

3.4.5. Aerobic Activity

To improve functional status and reduce pain, a program of aerobic activity, particularly aquatic program should be suggested to all patients with OA of the hip (ACR 1995 [2], OARSI 2008 [7], ACR 2010 [9]).

3.4.6. Manipulation and Stretching

Manipulation and stretching should be considered as an adjunct core treatment (NICE 2008 [8]). Manipulation is defined as high velocity thrusts.

3.5. Recommendations Specific for Hand OA

3.5.1. Patient Education

ACR 2010 recommendations suggests that all patients with hand OA should be evaluated for their ability to perform activities of daily living and receive instruction in joint protection techniques and the use of thermal agents for relief of pain and stiffness (ACR 2010[9]).

3.5.2. Splints and Orthoses

Patients with OA involving the trapeziometacarpal (1st carpometacarpal) joint may benefit from splinting (EULAR 2007 [6]; ACR 2010 [9]) and orthoses to prevent/correct lateral angulations and flexion deformity (EULAR 2007[6]). However, splint protection for thumb base OA may need to consider inclusion of a wrist component to increase the clinical effect (EULAR 2007 [6]).

3.5.3. Heat

Local application of heat (*e.g.* paraffin wax, hot pack) especially before exercises, and ultrasound are recommended by EULAR (EULAR 2007 [6]).

4. WHAT ARE THE MAIN DIFFERENCES BETWEEN THESE RECOMMENDATIONS?

4.1. Methodology

All the recommendations described herein are based on the best available evidence efficacy and safety of non-pharmacological modalities as well as the consensus judgment of clinical experts from different disciplines balancing the benefits and drawbacks of these therapies (Table **5**). However, it is evident that there are differences between the reviewed recommendations. For recommendations on hip and knee, the EULAR panel consisted of only rheumatologists and orthopaedic surgeons; for the hand OA recommendations, EULAR added a psychiatrist and two allied health professionals. The OARSI panel included two primary care physicians in addition to rheumatologists and an orthopaedic surgeon. By contrast, NICE and 2010 ACR experts panel included primary care physicians, physchiatrists, geriatrians, orthopaedic surgeons along with rheumatologists. NICE group is the only one expert group that integrates representatives from patients and physical therapists. The ACR expert panel had members from North America exclusively, EULAR group had only European members, NICE had only UK members and OARSI had representatives from Asia, Europe and US. Both EULAR and OARSI used modifications of the Delphi technique to generate lists of propositions. EULAR limited itself to a total of 11, 10 and 10 propositions for hand, hip and knee OA, respectively, while OARSI included 25 propositions in its recommendations for hip and knee OA. EULAR required 3, 3 and 5 rounds for the recommendations for hip, hand and knee OA respectively, while OARSI required six rounds to complete the Delphi exercises. In the development of hybrid guidelines by the EULAR OA task force, experts consensus on the most important propositions was followed by a systematic search for evidence, prior to assigning a strength and confidence of recommendation for each treatment. The sequence of steps has been modified slightly for the development of the OARSI treatment guidelines. An initial systematic review of evidence was followed by the development of expert consensus based on a combined consideration of the research evidence and the clinical expertise of the member committee. This was then followed by assignment of strength and confidence of recommendation for exact proposition as before. The 2010 ACR recommendations [9] were developed using a GRADE process, a comprehensive, explicit and transparent methodology, and do not include propositions; rather, the expert group used the best available evidence for the efficacy and safety of each modality to produce specific recommendations, either strong or weak or none, for the use of each modality relative to a specific clinical scenario. These scenarios included a base case of a patient with symptomatic hand, hip or knee OA.

4.2. Modalities

The critical appraisal of the EULAR, ACR2010, NICE and OARSI guidelines for hip and knee OA showed that few modalities are common to all recommendations (Table **6**). This core set of universally recommended modalities include weight loss, exercises and walking aids. Patient education and information are also recommended by EULAR, NICE and OARSI, but not by 2010 ACR. Patient education/information modality was recommended in the previous ACR recommendation but not the 2010 updated version.It was apparent that this core set of universally recommended therapies are all supported by strong evidence. Other modalities were addressed in only one or two recommendations whereas they were supported by a low level of evidence. These modalities include manipulation, regular phone contact, psychological intervention, referral to a physical therapist, insoles and ultrasound. This paradox is well illustrated in two of the OARSI recommendations. Walking aids and referral to a physical therapists had a level of evidence IV (expert committee reports or opinion or clinical experience of respected authorities, or both) but reach 100% of consensus and were strongly recommended (strength of the recommendations was 90%) the NICE, manipulation was recommended only on the basis of clinical expert opinion. Finally, there are some modalities which were evaluated by the experts but not recommended due to lack of evidence or experts consensus (Table **7**). This group included massage, isokinetic exercises, pulsed electromagnetic fields, Tai Chi, dietary therapies and laser. Somewhat surprising is the recommendation that patients be contacted regularly by phone in order to improve their clinical status. It rest on a single trial, whose randomized controlled design produced a high level of evidence. Few physician or even allied health professionals take time to call their patients in order to provide them with psychological support. Further, the majority are probably not appropriately skilled to manage this [16].

Table 5: Methods for developing recommendations.

	OARSI	EULAR	NICE	ACR
Targeted joint	Hip & knee	Hip or Knee or Hand	All joint (holistic approach)	Hand and knee and hip
Publication date	2008	2000, 2005, 2007	2008	2010
Methods	Systematic review Quality assessment Grading the evidence statement Formulation of the recommendations Delphi Strength of recommendation	Systematic review Quality assessment Grading the evidence statement	Developing evidence-based questions Systematic review Critical appraisal of the evidence Grading the evidence statement Formulating the recommendation Agreeing the recommendations	Systematic review Elaboration of clinical scenarios Quality assessment Formulation of the recommendations Grading strength of recommendations
Number of experts	16	21-23	18	13
Medical discipline of the experts	Primary care (2) Rheumatologists (11) Orthopedic surgeons (1) EBM (2)	Rheumatologist (16-19) Orthopedic surgeons (4) and/or Methodologists/Epidemiologist (2) and/or Allied health professional (1) and/or Physiatrist (1).	Rheumatologists (4), general practitioners (1), physiotherapists (2), geriatrist (1), medical statistician (1), health economist (1), epidemiologist (1), nurse (1), information scientist (1), health service research fellow (1), user-organization representative (2), vice-dean (1), clinical advisor (1)	Primary care physicians (4) Psychiatrists (1) Geritricians (1) Rheumatologists (2) Orthopaedic surgeon (1) Physical and occupational therapists (4)
Origin of the experts	USA, UK, Canada, France, Netherlands, Sweden.	European countries (12-14)	United Kingdom	USA, Canada

EBM = Evidence based medicine.

4.3. Limitations

Although the guidelines committees, except for NICE guidelines committee, are multinational some world areas are in general underrepresented. For example, the Asian population was not represented. 2010 ACR included only North America experts, EULAR only Europeans experts [17].

Only the NICE guideline expert group included allied health professions such as physiotherapy. In the other guidelines, allied health professions were not represented despite the majority of the formulated recommendations concerning non-pharmacological modalities. Conceivably, the recommendations on non-pharmacological modalities might have been very different if they had been developed by a panel of experts composed only of physical therapists.

With the exception of NICE guidelines, patient's perspectives on the recommendations remain unknown. Their perspective is important to determine acceptability and to facilitate adherence.

Table 6: Non-pharmacologic therapies recommended for patients with osteoarthritis.

ACR 2010	EULAR	OARSI	NICE
Hip	**Hip**	**Hip**	**For all OA**
• Cardiovascular and resistance land-based exercises. • Aquatic exercises • Weight loss • Participation in self-management programs. • Manual therapy in combination with supervised exercises. • Psychological interventions. • Thermal agents • Walking aids	• Patient education • Exercises • Appliance (Sticks, insoles). • Weight reduction	• Patient education and information • Referral to a physical therapist • Regular phone contact • TENS • Heat/cold therapy • Walking aids/frames or wheeled walkers for bilateral disease • Advise about footwear • Weight reduction • Exercises • Exercises in water	• Patient information • Self-management strategies/programmes. • Heat/cold therapy • Exercises strengthening/aerobic fitness • Manipulation • Stretching • Weight loss • Ultrasound • Footwear • Bracing/insoles/joint support • Assistive devices
Knee	**Knee**	**Knee**	
• Cardiovascular and resistance land-based exercise • Aquatic exercise • Weight loss • Self-management programs • Psychological interventions • Medially directed patellar taping. • Wedged insoles • Thermal agents • Walking aids • Acupuncture • TENS	• Patient education • Exercises • Appliances (sticks, insoles, knee bracing) • Weight reduction	• Patient education and information • Referral to a physical therapist • Regular phone contact • TENS • Heat/cold therapy • Walking aids/frames or wheeled walkers for bilateral disease • Weight reduction • Acupuncture • Advice about footwear • Insoles/lateral wedge insoles • Knee bracing • Exercises	
Hand	**Hand**	**Hand**	
• Evaluation of ADL • Instruction of joint protection techniques • Assistive devices • Instruction in use of thermal modalities • Splints	• Patient education • Exercises • Local heat • Ultrasound • Splint/orthoses for thumb	• None	

TENS = Transcutaneous Electrical nerve Stimulation; ADL = Activities of Daily Living.

Some of the recommendations for non-pharmacological treatments are simple common sense. They stem chiefly from expert opinion, often with little objective evidence to support them. Examples include referral to a physical therapist, and regular exercise.

Recommendations about non-pharmacological treatments raise the issue of the placebo or the comparative therapy. In general, the tested modality is compared to sham therapy, waiting list, no treatment or current pharmacological treatments.

In contrast, some modalities including TENS or acupuncture with a high level of evidence (Ia) were weakly or not recommended. TENS was recommended only by OARSI and manipulation only by NICE. In OARSI guidelines, TENS had a high level of evidence but a mitigate level of consensus (69 %) and the strength of the recommendation was low (59%).

5. HOW ARE THESE RECOMMENDATIONS USED IN CLINICAL PRACTICE?

Overall, recommendations are useful. They provide an opportunity to update clinical practice as new treatments become available, based on the experience acquired by international experts. Improvements in patient care are seen in several areas of clinical practice when guidelines are properly followed. The development and publication of guidelines is a necessary, but not a sufficient step for introducing evidence-based practice to the clinical management of patients. In fact, one-third of patient with OA fail to receive recommended care. A pilot survey of the perceived usefulness of the treatment modalities addressed by the existing guidelines was conducted among physicians and other health care professionals attending the New York University-OARSI Rheumatology Symposium in 2006. The purpose of the survey was to collect the user opinions on the usefulness of current treatment guidelines. Of the 19 participants who completed the questionnaire, more than 70% perceived combination therapy to be very useful or essential for knee and hip OA management. Weight reduction was perceived to be more useful for knee than hip OA by 68%, whereas self-management, exercise and education were considered useful for both hip and knee OA. An Italian survey clearly demonstrates that only 41% of the general practitioners concomitantly use pharmacological and non-pharmacological modalities whereas this approach is systematically recommended [18]. The large majority of patients were managed by general practitioners in primary care with analgesic or non-steroidal anti-inflammatory drugs to relieve pain. In the UK, the recommendations of exercise, patient education and self-management (NICE) are usually observed by physiotherapists, but other modalities such as ultrasound and pulsed short-wave are often used despite the lack of or poor research evidence supporting their efficiency [19]. Another survey has reported disparities between physical therapists' current use of therapeutic exercise for knee OA and the recent MOVE recommendations in term of type of exercises prescribed and the delivery of exercises [20]. These recent studies clearly illustrate the difficulties in implementing clinical practice guidelines into practice.

The following factors have been identified as major factors that influence physician adoption of clinical practice guidelines [17]: (1) lack of awareness of gaps in quality of care for people with OA, (2) the lack of prioritization of OA compared to other inflammatory rheumatic conditions, (3) the difficulty in accessing this knowledge (lack of time, language problems, etc), (4) an inadequate training in the theory and practice of quality improvement methods, in qualitative evaluation methods and in project management, (5) the difficulty in applying the guidelines in the practitioners' daily practice (inflexible, oversimplified, reluctance for change, lack of agreement, the lack of outcome expectancy), (6) lack of adaptation of knowledge to the local environment of the health care system (health care policy, drug reimbursement, local habits etc), (7) the lack of systems to support ongoing review and updating of evidence based recommendations.

Recently, Brand [21] has proposed strategies and enablers for translating evidence into practice for people with OA of the hip and knee. Among the strategies and enablers identified by this author, the most important were: evidence-based recommendation summary tables, checklist recommendation reminder sheet, involvement of clinician leaders, peer review and scientific meeting presentations, audit and feedback of new evidence-based practice, patient satisfaction assessment, and a goal setting care template for health professionals.

CONCLUDING REMARKS

Numerous non-pharmacological modalities are commonly recommended by the most popular medical and scientific societies specialized in the field of OA. The majority of these recommendations are based on experimental evidence and/or strong expert conviction. The core treatments that should be considered for every person with OA are education, information access, and aerobic and strengthening exercises. However, in a large number of countries, these modalities are not considered as a first line treatment but rather as an alternative to pharmacological treatments in patients with co-morbidities.

Table 7: Non-pharmacologic therapies evaluated but not recommended for patients with osteoarthritis*.

ACR	EULAR	OARSI	NICE
Hip	**Hip**	**Hip**	**For all OA**
• Dietary therapy and other unproven therapies (2005) • Balance exercises, either alone or in combination with strengthening exercises • Tai chi • Manual therapy alone	• Acupuncture • Spa/Sauna	• Ultrasound • Laser • Massage • Acupuncture	• Rest • Relaxing • Pacing • Massage • Hydrotherapy • Tai chi • Aquatic exercise • Isokinetic • Ultrasound • Pulsed electromagnetic field • Interferential therapy • Laser • Acupuncture
Knee	**Knee**	**Knee**	
• Specific dietary therapy and other unproven therapies (2005) • Balance exercises, either alone or in combination with strengthening exercises. • Tai chi • Laterally wedged insoles • Manual therapy alone • Braces • Laterally directed patellar taping	• Laser • Spa • Pulsed EMF • Ultrasound • TENS • Acupuncture	• Ultrasound • Laser • Massage • Self-management	
Hand	**Hand**	**Hand**	
• None	• Laser • TENS	• None	

*These modalities have been studied but not recommended because there is a lack of evidence of their efficacy, or a higher risk/benefit ratio, or a higher economical impact.

One reason is that medical doctors are not convinced by the efficacy of non-pharmacological treatment, probably because some of them lack clinical evidence. Another reason is that patients are waiting for passive treatment, and that it may be difficult to obtain patients' participation in an active treatment. Additional data are required to support the key role played by non-pharmacological treatments in the algorithm of OA management and to demonstrate their superiority in term of cost/benefit ratio. For example, in low back pain, manipulation is not more efficient than standard pharmacological treatment (acetaminophen, NSAIDs) but its economic impact is less. Further, non-pharmacological treatments are generally safe, suggesting their suitability for long-term application in elderly people with co-morbidities. Even when there is a lack of clinical evidence of their efficacy, non-pharmacological modalities should be considered as a first line treatment to decrease drug consumption, to relief pain and to reduce disability in OA patients.

REFERENCES

[1] Zhang W, Moskowitz RW, Nuki G, *et al.* OARSI recommendations for the management of hip and knee osteoarthritis, part I: critical appraisal of existing treatment guidelines and systematic review of current research evidence. Osteoarthritis Cartilage 2007; 15: 981-1000.

[2] Hochberg MC, Altman RD, Brandt KD, *et al.* Guidelines for the medical management of osteoarthritis. Part I. Osteoarthritis of the hip. American College of Rheumatology. Arthritis Rheum 1995; 38: 1535-40.

[3] Hochberg MC, Altman RD, Brandt KD, *et al.* Guidelines for the medical management of osteoarthritis. Part II. Osteoarthritis of the knee. American College of Rheumatology. Arthritis Rheum 1995; 38: 1541-6.

[4] Zhang W, Doherty M, Arden N, *et al.* EULAR evidence based recommendations for the management of hip osteoarthritis: report of a task force of the EULAR Standing Committee for International Clinical Studies Including Therapeutics (ESCISIT). Ann Rheum Dis 2005; 64: 669-81.

[5] Zhang W, Doherty M. EULAR recommendations for knee and hip osteoarthritis: a critique of the methodology. Br J Sports Med 2006; 40: 664-9.

[6] Zhang W, Doherty M, Leeb BF, *et al.* EULAR evidence-based recommendations for the diagnosis of hand osteoarthritis: report of a task force of ESCISIT. Ann Rheum Dis 2007; 68: 8-17.

[7] Zhang W, Moskowitz RW, Nuki G, *et al.* OARSI recommendations for the management of hip and knee osteoarthritis, Part II: OARSI evidence-based, expert consensus guidelines. Osteoarthritis Cartilage 2008; 16: 137-62.

[8] National Institute for health and Clinical Excellence. Osteoarthritis: national clinical guideline for care and management in adults. London: NICE wwwniceorguk/CG059 2008.

[9] Hochberg M, Altman R, Benkhalti M, *et al.* The 2010 American College of Rheumatology Recommendations for Non-Pharmacologic and Pharmacologic Therapies in Hand, Hip and Knee Osteoarthritis. Arthritis Care Res 2010; Submitted.

[10] Henrotin Y, Sanchez C, Balligand M. Pharmaceutical and nutraceutical management of canine osteoarthritis: present and future perspectives. Vet J 2005; 170: 113-23.

[11] Ameye LG, Chee WS. Osteoarthritis and nutrition. From nutraceuticals to functional foods: a systematic review of the scientific evidence. Arthritis Res Ther 2006; 8: R127.

[12] Atkins D, Best D, Briss PA, *et al.* Grading quality of evidence and strength of recommendations. BMJ 2004; 328: 1490.

[13] Pendleton A, Arden N, Dougados M, *et al.* EULAR recommendations for the management of knee osteoarthritis: report of a task force of the Standing Committee for International Clinical Studies Including Therapeutic Trials (ESCISIT). Ann Rheum Dis 2000; 59: 936-44.

[14] Jordan KM, Arden NK, Doherty M, *et al.* EULAR Recommendations 2003: an evidence based approach to the management of knee osteoarthritis: Report of a Task Force of the Standing Committee for International Clinical Studies Including Therapeutic Trials (ESCISIT). Ann Rheum Dis 2003; 62: 1145-55.

[15] Recommendations for the medical management of osteoarthritis of the hip and knee. 2000 update. American College of Rheumatology subcommittee on osteoarthritis guidelines. Arthritis Rheum 2000; 43: 1905-15.

[16] Chevalier X, Henrotin Y. OARSI recommendations on knee and hip osteoarthritis: use with discernment. Joint Bone Spine 2009; 76: 455-7.

[17] Henrotin Y. Need for high-standard translation methodology for the dissemination of guidelines. Osteoarthritis Cartilage 2009;17:1536-8.

[18] Sarzi-Puttini P, Cimmino MA, Scarpa R, *et al.* Do physicians treat symptomatic osteoarthritis patients properly? Results of the AMICA experience. Semin Arthritis Rheum 2005; 35: 38-42.

[19] Walsh NE, Hurley MV. Evidence based guidelines and current practice for physiotherapy management of knee osteoarthritis. Musculoskeletal Care 2009; 7: 45-56.

[20] Holden MA, Nicholls EE, Hay EM, *et al.* Physical therapists' use of therapeutic exercise for patients with clinical knee osteoarthritis in the United kingdom: in line with current recommendations? Phys Ther 2008; 88: 1109-21.

[21] Brand C, Cox S. Systems for implementing best practice for a chronic disease: management of osteoarthritis of the hip and knee. Intern Med J 2006; 36: 170-9.

CHAPTER 4

Weight Loss: Preventive and Therapeutic Effects in Obese Patients with Osteoarthritis

P. Richette[*]

Université Paris 7, UFR médicale, Assistance Publique-Hôpitaux de Paris, Hôpital Lariboisière, Fédération de Rhumatologie, 75475 Paris Cedex 10, France

Abstract: Obesity is the most modifiable risk factor for knee Osteoarthritis (OA). The mechanisms by which obesity contributes to the onset of knee OA are not fully understood, but the increase in biomechanical loading to cartilage seems to play a major role. Recent data have also suggested that metabolic factors and low-grade inflammation in obese patients might contribute to the genesis of the OA process. Weight loss is recommended by international bodies (EULAR and OARSI) as a treatment modality for obese patients with knee OA. RCTs have demonstrated that moderate dietary weight loss of about 5% improves function but pain only slightly. Few open studies have investigated the effect of massive weight loss induced by bariatric surgery in knee OA. Although the results from these studies should be cautiously interpreted, it seems that drastic weight loss could be more effective to reduce pain and disability in obese patients. Moderate weight loss significantly reduces several markers of systemic inflammation (TNFα, IL-6 and CRP) but the search for a correlation between these changes and an improvement in clinical outcomes has remained elusive in different studies.

Keywords: Osteoarthritis, obesity, weight loss, adipokines, inflammation.

1. OBESITY AND OSTEOARTHRITIS

Obesity is a major concern in Europe, North America and other developed countries. In fact, obesity now affects almost two thirds of Americans [1]. In Europe, the prevalence of obesity seems lower but recent epidemiological studies have shown in some countries a sharp increase in its prevalence since a decade [2, 3]. Among all the co-morbidities related to obesity in males, type II diabetes and osteoarthritis (OA) were recently shown to be the most frequent [4].

It has been demonstrated that the risk for OA of the knee was increased almost four-fold in obese women and 4.8-fold in obese men whose body mass index (BMI) was in the range 30–35 compared with those whose BMI was < 25 in the first National Health and Nutrition Examination survey. The risk for OA of the knee is increased by approximately 15% for each additional unit increase in BMI > 27 [5].

Obesity is thus the main modifiable risk factor for the onset of knee OA [6], and some work, but not all [7], have also suggested that obesity might increase the risk of structural progression in knees with pre-existing OA [8, 9]. The strong association between BMI and OA of the knee is thought to be mainly due to an increase in mechanical loads to the tibio-femoral cartilage. Indeed, chondrocytes express several mechanoreceptors (CD44, α5β1 integrins, stretch-activated channels) [10], in whom activation triggers cascades of intracellular events which lead to the production of deleterious mediators and thus to the degradation of the extracellular matrix [11].

The observation that obesity is also a risk factor for non-bearing joints such as hand OA [12] have raised the hypothesis that the link between overweight and OA could also occur through systemic inflammation, where the adipose tissue would act as an endocrine organ releasing in blood several pro inflammatory mediators and adipokines, participating in cartilage alteration in obese [13-16]. With obesity and insulin resistance, adipose tissue contains many macrophages and secretes inflammatory cytokines such as Interleukin-6 (IL-6), Tumor

*Address correspondence to P. Richette: Fédération de Rhumatologie, Hôpital Lariboisière, 2 Rue Ambroise Paré, 75475 Paris cedex 10, France; Tel: + 33- 1-49-95-62-90; Fax: + 33- 1 49-95-86-31; E-mail: pascal.richette@lrb.aphp.fr

Necrosis Factor (TNF) α, serum-amyloid A, and high levels of leptin, resistin and visfatin and low levels of adiponectin [17-19]. *In vitro* and *in vivo* studies have shown that all these adipokines could impact cartilage homeostasis [20-23]. Additionally, besides the possible involvement of inflammatory cytokines and adipokines in the pathogenesis of OA in obese patients, some studies have suggested that metabolic risk factors such as diabetes mellitus, triglycerides and cholesterols levels might also be associated with OA [24, 25].

2. EFFECTS OF MODERATE WEIGHT LOSS ON SYMPTOMS IN PATIENTS WITH PRE-EXISTING KNEE OA

Obesity clearly increases the incidence of knee OA, obviously through an increase in mechanical cartilage stress and perhaps also through systemic effects. It has been shown that each pound of weight loss results in a four-fold reduction in the load of the knee per step during daily activities [26]. However, loss of muscle mass has been a subject of concern in weight-loss programs given the important shock absorbing and stabilising roles of muscles. The effect of a 6-month intentional weight loss program combined with exercises on muscle strength has been investigated in older obese adults with knee OA. It was found that changes in lean body mass and fat mass were inversely associated with changes in muscle strength and quality measures [27].

But can weight loss reduce pain and disability in patients with knee OA? Although weight reduction is a treatment modality in obese patients with knee OA according to the EULAR and OARSI recommendations [28, 29], few therapeutic trials have specifically examined the effect of moderate weight loss in OA of the knee [30-33]. There are two good quality Randomized Controlled Trials (RCT)s [30, 31] that have assessed the effect of weight reduction on pain and disability as outcomes in knee OA patients. The Arthritis, Diet and Activity Promotion Trial (ADAPT) was an 18-month single blind randomized clinical trial designed to determine if exercise and dietary weight loss, alone or in combination, were more effective than usual care in improving pain and function in older overweight and obese adults with knee OA. The diet groups achieved 5% weight loss over 18 months using a reduced-calorie diet with behavioural strategies [31]. Using an intensive low-energy diet, obese patients enrolled in the study performed by Christensen *et al.* lost a mean of 11% BMI over an 8 weeks period, as compared to patients in the control group who lost a mean of 4.3 % [30]. Using data from these two RCTs, Zhang *et al.* found that the Effect Sizes (ES)s for relief of pain (ES=0.13, 95%CI -0.12, 0.38), stiffness (0.36 95% CI -0.08, 0.80) and functional improvement (0.69 95% CI 0.24, 1.14) were small to moderate with an number-needed-to-treat of 3 (95% CI 2, 9) for a decrease in WOMAC scores of >50%, 8 weeks after commencing a low energy diet (3.4 MJ/day) [29].

A systematic review and meta-analysis of four RCTs with data on 454 obese patients with knee OA has been performed by Christensen *et al.* The pooled ESs for improvements in pain and physical disability are small (ES=0.20 95% CI 0, 0.39 and ES=0.23 95% CI 0.04, 0.42, respectively), with a mean weight reduction of 6.1 kg (range 4.7 to 7.6 kg). Meta-regression analysis demonstrated significant improvement in disability with weight loss > 5% or at a rate of >0.24%/week (Table 1) [34]. Taken together, these data suggest that moderate weight loss improves function, and pain slightly in knee OA. There are no published RCTs to confirm comparable benefits from weight loss in patients with hip OA.

Table 1. Interventions leading to weight loss versus control in obese patients with knee osteoarthritis. Adapted from [43].

Outcomes at 6 weeks to 18 months	Number of trials [30-33]	Mean difference in weight loss between groups (95% CI)	Weighted effect size(ES)† (CI)
Pain	4	6.1 kg (4.7 to 7.6)	0.20 (0 to 0.39)‡
Self-reported disability	4	6.1 kg (4.7 to 7.6)	0.23 (0.04 to 0.42)§
Patient global evaluation (Lequesne Index)	2	4.7 kg (4.0 to 5.5)	0.58 (−0.4 to 1.56)‡¶

*Analysis based on a fixed-effects model, † Standardised mean difference, ‡ Not significant.

§ Favours weight loss, ¶Based on a random-effects model.

3. EFFECT OF MASSIVE WEIGHT LOSS ON PAIN AND FUNCTION IN OBESE PATIENTS WITH KNEE OA

A small number of studies have investigated the effect of massive weight loss following bariatric surgery in patients with knee OA [35, 36]. Bariatric surgical techniques include mainly gastric bypass and laparoscopic adjustable gastric banding [37]. Criteria for obesity surgery are BMI $\geq$ 40 kg/m^2 or $\geq$ 35 kg/m^2 with at least one co-morbidity (hypertension, diabetes mellitus, dyslipidemia, obstructive sleep apnea syndrome) [37]. In the most recent uncontrolled study, 44 obese patients were assessed for different musculoskeletal conditions before and after surgery. The mean time from surgery to the follow-up visit was 201+/-50 days and the mean BMIs pre-operation and post-operation were 51+/-8 and 54 +/-9, respectively. Among the 44 patients, 32 complained of knee pain and met the American College of Rheumatology (ACR) criteria for knee OA. In these patients, the WOMAC total score significantly decreased from 150+/-75.4 mm to 49+/-51 mm (absolute change 67%, P<0.001). The different WOMAC subscores for pain (51%), function (74%) and stiffness (64%) were also significantly improved (P<0.001 for each). In another open study, measurements of the Joint Space Width (JSW) of the knee by digital image computer were performed before and after surgically-induced weight loss in 64 obese patients. During 8-months period, a significant reduction in BMI was observed in the study group, from 43.3 to 37.0. For both men and women, the minimal medial JSW for the right knee increased, on average, by 0.7 mm (P<0.001). Pain and function, as assessed by the American Knee Society Score (KSS), were greatly improved (P<0.001) [35].

Although the design of these studies does not allow definitive conclusions to be drawn, their results suggest that massive weight loss alleviates both pain and function. This model of bariatric surgery is of great interest to explore whether the beneficial effects of weight loss on symptoms in patients with knee OA might occur through systemic modifications, because this surgery results in important metabolic changes that lead to major improvements in blood glucose and insulin levels, insulin sensitivity and hormonal responses, as well as decreasing inflammatory markers [38]. To our knowledge, no such study has been conducted.

4. EFFECTS OF MODERATE WEIGHT LOSS ON BIOCHEMICAL MARKERS

Chua *et al.* have determined the correlation of selected joint biomarkers with clinical outcome measures in an intervention study using serum samples collected from participants in the Arthritis, Diet, and Activity Promotion Trial (ADAPT) [31]. The biomarkers were the Cartilage Oligomeric Matrix Protein (COMP), hyaluronan (HA), antigenic keratan sulphate (AgKS) epitopes and transforming growth factor- β 1 (TGF-β1). The biomarker levels remained relatively stable during the 18 months of the study, except for AgKS which slightly decreased, and any differences observed between intervention groups were quite minimal. The authors found only weak correlations with change in AgKS (P=0.03) and COMP (P=0.02) and change in weight over 18 months. In other studies using serum samples from the ADAPT subjects, it has been shown that the dietary weight loss but not the exercise intervention significantly reduced levels of the inflammation markers, C-reactive protein, IL-6, and soluble tumor necrosis factor alpha receptor 1, and reduced the levels of the leptin [39, 40]. Conversely, Miller *et al.* found that weight loss approaching 10 % over 6 months in older obese patients with knee OA produced minor effects on inflammatory markers (IL-6, TNF alpha, CRP, sTNFR1 and sTNFR2). Furthermore, there were weak correlations between measures of physical function and inflammatory markers. Thus, these studies provided inconclusive results on the effect of moderate weight loss on joint biomarkers, and on the correlations between improvement in inflammatory markers and clinical outcomes for knee OA.

5. EFFECT OF WEIGHT LOSS IN PRIMARY PREVENTION

The Framingham study has shown that a decrease in BMI of >2 units in women over the previous 10 years decreased the odds of developing OA of the knee by over 50% (OR= 0.46, 95% CI 0.24 to 0.86). The risk of OA of the knee in women with increased baseline BMI also decreased by almost 60% with >2 units of BMI loss. In women free of disease at baseline, a higher BMI increased the risk of OA (OR 1.6 (per 5-unit increase), 95% CI 1.2 to 2.2), and weight change was directly correlated with risk of OA (OR 1.4 (per 10-

pound change in weight), 95%CI 1.1 to 1.8) [3, 41]. Finally, Felson *et al.* have computed that eliminating obesity in USA could itself prevent anywhere from 25.1% to 48.3% of knee OA in women, and from 26.6% to 51.8% in men [42].

6. CONCLUDING REMARKS

Obesity is a powerful risk factor for the development of knee OA. Given that obesity is associated with the onset and possibly progression of OA, weight loss represents an important preventive strategy. There is good evidence to support that moderate weight loss improves function in obese patients with pre-existing knee OA.

REFERENCES

[1]   Flegal KM, Carroll MD, Ogden CL, Curtin LR. Prevalence and trends in obesity among US adults, 1999-2008. Jama 2010; 303(3): 235-41.

[2]   Charles MA, Eschwege E, Basdevant A. Monitoring the obesity epidemic in France: the Obepi surveys 1997-2006. Obesity (Silver Spring) 2008; 16(9): 2182-6.

[3]   Woolf AD, Breedveld F, Kvien TK. Controlling the obesity epidemic is important for maintaining musculoskeletal health. Ann Rheum Dis 2006; 65(11):1401-2.

[4]   Guh DP, Zhang W, Bansback N, Amarsi Z, Birmingham CL, Anis AH. The incidence of co-morbidities related to obesity and overweight: a systematic review and meta-analysis. BMC Public Health 2009; 9: 88.

[5]   Anderson JJ, Felson DT. Factors associated with osteoarthritis of the knee in the first national Health and Nutrition Examination Survey (HANES I). Evidence for an association with overweight, race, and physical demands of work. Am J Epidemiol 1988; 128(1): 179-89.

[6]   Blagojevic M, Jinks C, Jeffery A, Jordan KP. Risk factors for onset of osteoarthritis of the knee in older adults: a systematic review and meta-analysis. Osteoarthritis Cartilage 2009;18: 24-33.

[7]   Le Graverand MP, Brandt K, Mazzuca SA, Raunig D, Vignon E. Progressive increase in body mass index is not associated with a progressive increase in joint space narrowing in obese women with osteoarthritis of the knee. Ann Rheum Dis 2009; 68(11): 1734-8.

[8]   Niu J, Zhang YQ, Torner J, *et al.* Is obesity a risk factor for progressive radiographic knee osteoarthritis? Arthritis Rheum 2009; 61(3): 329-35.

[9]   Reijman M, Pols HA, Bergink AP, *et al.* Body mass index associated with onset and progression of osteoarthritis of the knee but not of the hip: the Rotterdam Study. Ann Rheum Dis 2007; 66(2): 158-62.

[10]   Mobasheri A, Carter SD, Martin-Vasallo P, Shakibaei M. Integrins and stretch activated ion channels; putative components of functional cell surface mechanoreceptors in articular chondrocytes. Cell Biol Int 2002; 26(1):1-18.

[11]   Pottie P, Presle N, Terlain B, Netter P, Mainard D, Berenbaum F. Obesity and osteoarthritis: more complex than predicted! Ann Rheum Dis 2006; 65(11): 1403-5.

[12]   Yusuf E, Nelissen R, Ioan-Facsinay A, *et al.* Association between weight or Body Mass Index and hand osteoarthritis: a systematic review. Ann Rheum Dis 2009.

[13]   Abramson SB, Attur M. Developments in the scientific understanding of osteoarthritis. Arthritis Res Ther 2009; 11(3): 227.

[14]   Messier SP. Obesity and osteoarthritis: disease genesis and nonpharmacologic weight management. Rheum Dis Clin North Am 2008; 34(3): 713-29.

[15]   Griffin TM, Guilak F. Why is obesity associated with osteoarthritis? Insights from mouse models of obesity. Biorheology 2008; 45(3-4): 387-98.

[16]   Sandell LJ. Obesity and osteoarthritis: is leptin the link? Arthritis Rheum 2009;60(10):2858-60.

[17]   Rasouli N, Kern PA. Adipocytokines and the metabolic complications of obesity. J Clin Endocrinol Metab 2008; 93(11 Suppl 1):S64-73.

[18]   Poitou C, Coussieu C, Rouault C, *et al.* Serum amyloid A: a marker of adiposity-induced low-grade inflammation but not of metabolic status. Obesity (Silver Spring) 2006; 14(2):309-18.

[19]   Henegar C, Tordjman J, Achard V, *et al.* Adipose tissue transcriptomic signature highlights the pathological relevance of extracellular matrix in human obesity. Genome Biol 2008; 9(1): R14.

[20]   Gomez R, Lago F, Gomez-Reino J, Dieguez C, Gualillo O. Adipokines in the skeleton: influence on cartilage function and joint degenerative diseases. J Mol Endocrinol 2009; 43(1): 11-8.

[21]   Griffin TM, Huebner JL, Kraus VB, Guilak F. Extreme obesity due to impaired leptin signaling in mice does not cause knee osteoarthritis. Arthritis Rheum 2009; 60(10): 2935-44.

[22]   Lee JH, Ort T, Ma K, *et al.* Resistin is elevated following traumatic joint injury and causes matrix degradation and release of inflammatory cytokines from articular cartilage *in vitro*. Osteoarthritis Cartilage 2009; 17(5): 613-20.

[23]   Gosset M, Berenbaum F, Salvat C, *et al.* Crucial role of visfatin/pre-B cell colony-enhancing factor in matrix degradation and prostaglandin E2 synthesis in chondrocytes: possible influence on osteoarthritis. Arthritis Rheum 2008; 58(5): 1399-409.

[24]   Sowers M, Karvonen-Gutierrez CA, Palmieri-Smith R, Jacobson JA, Jiang Y, Ashton-Miller JA. Knee osteoarthritis in obese women with cardiometabolic clustering. Arthritis Rheum 2009; 61(10): 1328-36.

[25]   Hart DJ, Doyle DV, Spector TD. Association between metabolic factors and knee osteoarthritis in women: the Chingford Study. J Rheumatol 1995; 22(6): 1118-23.

[26]   Messier SP, Gutekunst DJ, Davis C, DeVita P. Weight loss reduces knee-joint loads in overweight and obese older adults with knee osteoarthritis. Arthritis Rheum 2005; 52(7): 2026-32.

[27]   Wang X, Miller GD, Messier SP, Nicklas BJ. Knee strength maintained despite loss of lean body mass during weight loss in older obese adults with knee osteoarthritis. J Gerontol A Biol Sci Med Sci 2007; 62(8): 866-71.

[28]   Jordan KM, Arden NK, Doherty M, *et al.* EULAR Recommendations 2003: an evidence based approach to the management of knee osteoarthritis: Report of a Task Force of the Standing Committee for International Clinical Studies Including Therapeutic Trials (ESCISIT). Ann Rheum Dis 2003; 62(12): 1145-55.

[29]   Zhang W, Moskowitz RW, Nuki G, et al. OARSI recommendations for the management of hip and knee osteoarthritis, Part II: OARSI evidence-based, expert consensus guidelines. Osteoarthritis Cartilage 2008; 16(2): 137-62.

[30]   Christensen R, Astrup A, Bliddal H. Weight loss: the treatment of choice for knee osteoarthritis? A randomized trial. Osteoarthritis Cartilage 2005; 13(1): 20-7.

[31]   Messier SP, Loeser RF, Miller GD, *et al.* Exercise and dietary weight loss in overweight and obese older adults with knee osteoarthritis: the Arthritis, Diet, and Activity Promotion Trial. Arthritis Rheum 2004; 50(5): 1501-10.

[32]   Messier SP, Loeser RF, Mitchell MN, *et al.* Exercise and weight loss in obese older adults with knee osteoarthritis: a preliminary study. J Am Geriatr Soc 2000; 48(9): 1062-72.

[33]   Toda Y, Toda T, Takemura S, Wada T, Morimoto T, Ogawa R. Change in body fat, but not body weight or metabolic correlates of obesity, is related to symptomatic relief of obese patients with knee osteoarthritis after a weight control program. J Rheumatol 1998; 25(11): 2181-6.

[34]   Christensen R, Bartels EM, Astrup A, Bliddal H. Effect of weight reduction in obese patients diagnosed with knee osteoarthritis: a systematic review and meta-analysis. Ann Rheum Dis 2007; 66(4): 433-9.

[35]   Abu-Abeid S, Wishnitzer N, Szold A, Liebergall M, Manor O. The influence of surgically-induced weight loss on the knee joint. Obes Surg 2005; 15(10): 1437-42.

[36]   Hooper MM, Stellato TA, Hallowell PT, Seitz BA, Moskowitz RW. Musculoskeletal findings in obese subjects before and after weight loss following bariatric surgery. Int J Obes (Lond) 2007; 31(1): 114-20.

[37]   Elder KA, Wolfe BM. Bariatric surgery: a review of procedures and outcomes. Gastroenterology 2007; 132(6): 2253-71.

[38]   Mutch DM, Fuhrmann JC, Rein D, *et al.* Metabolite profiling identifies candidate markers reflecting the clinical adaptations associated with Roux-en-Y gastric bypass surgery. PLoS One 2009; 4(11): e7905.

[39]   Nicklas BJ, Ambrosius W, Messier SP, *et al.* Diet-induced weight loss, exercise, and chronic inflammation in older, obese adults: a randomized controlled clinical trial. Am J Clin Nutr 2004; 79(4): 544-51.

[40]   Miller GD, Nicklas BJ, Davis CC, Ambrosius WT, Loeser RF, Messier SP. Is serum leptin related to physical function and is it modifiable through weight loss and exercise in older adults with knee osteoarthritis? Int J Obes Relat Metab Disord 2004; 28(11): 1383-90.

[41]   Felson DT, Zhang Y, Anthony JM, Naimark A, Anderson JJ. Weight loss reduces the risk for symptomatic knee osteoarthritis in women. The Framingham Study. Ann Intern Med 1992; 116(7): 535-9.

[42]   Felson DT, Zhang Y. An update on the epidemiology of knee and hip osteoarthritis with a view to prevention. Arthritis Rheum 1998; 41(8): 1343-55.

[43]   Ciliska D. Review: moderate weight loss reduces functional disability but does not reduce pain in obese patients with knee osteoarthritis. Evid Based Nurs 2008; 11(1):17.

CHAPTER 5

The Role of Land-Based Exercise and Manual Therapy in the Management of Osteoarthritis

K. Bennell[1*], M. Hunt[2] and R. Hinman[1]

[1] Centre for Health, Exercise & Sports Medicine, Department of Physiotherapy, School of Health Sciences, University of Melbourne, Melbourne, VIC, Australia and [2] Department of Physical Therapy, University of British Columbia, Vancouver, Canada

Abstract: This chapter covers the role of two commonly used modalities, land-based exercise and manual therapy, in the management of OA. It summarises available evidence for the effectiveness of these modalities and discusses practical issues related to their application in the clinical setting. Exercise is the cornerstone of management for OA and is recommended by all clinical guidelines. There is strong evidence to show short-term beneficial effects of exercise on pain and function for knee OA. While the type of exercise does not seem to influence treatment outcome, a combination of strengthening, aerobic and functional exercise is recommended. As therapist contact appears to improve outcomes, a period of supervised exercise delivered either individually or in a group setting followed by a home program may be most appropriate. Strategies to facilitate long-term adherence to exercise are needed given that the benefits of exercise decline over time principally due to a lack of adherence. Given the limited research into the effects of exercise for hip and hand OA, further studies are needed at these sites. Manual therapy is delivered by health practitioners from a range of disciplines and may include techniques such as manipulation, mobilisation, stretching, myofascial techniques and massage. Limited research suggests that manual therapy techniques may be beneficial in the management of large joint OA particularly at the hip and as an adjunct to core treatment strategies of exercise and education. No studies have investigated the effects of manual therapy techniques, other than massage, for OA of the hand so the benefits for this patient group are largely unknown.

Keywords: Osteoarthritis, exercises, manual therapy.

1. INTRODUCTION

This chapter will cover the role of two commonly used modalities, land-based exercise and manual therapy, in the management of Osteoarthritis (OA). It will summarise available evidence for the effectiveness of these modalities and discuss practical issues related to their application in the clinical setting. While there is a considerable amount of research into exercise, most is directed at knee OA with much less attention paid to the effects of exercise in individuals with hip and hand OA. Manual therapy is delivered by health practitioners from a range of disciplines but its role in OA has not been well studied.

2. LAND-BASED EXERCISE

Exercise is the cornerstone of OA management and is recommended by clinical guidelines [1, 2]. It can take many forms including: muscle strengthening, stretching/range of motion, aerobic conditioning, neuromuscular/balance and Tai Chi. Exercise dosage can vary in terms of frequency, intensity and duration. Additionally, the exercise can involve expensive, specialized equipment, or no equipment at all, and can be delivered in a group setting or individually. The nature of the exercise program will likely depend on patient-specific factors such as disease characteristics, goals of treatment, patient preference, resources and availability of equipment.

Exercise for individuals with OA has great potential to reduce symptoms and improve physical functioning.

*Address correspondence to K. Bennell: Centre for Health, Exercise & Sports Medicine, Department of Physiotherapy, School of Health Sciences, University of Melbourne, Melbourne, VIC, Australia, 3010; Tel: +61 3 8344 4171; Fax: +61 3 8344 4188; E-mail: k.bennell@unimelb.edu.au

Yves Henrotin, Kim Bennell and Francois Rannou (Eds)

Importantly, exercise is accompanied by few contraindications or adverse effects unlike drugs and surgery [3]. Exercise aims to address physical impairments associated with OA and typical physiological changes following exercise may include improvements in muscle strength, neuromuscular control, range of motion, joint stability and fitness. In addition to the potential for symptom reduction and functional gains, benefits for the overall health and well-being of the patient with exercise are also likely to be important. Although recent meta-analyses have found that the effects of exercise on psychological parameters in people with OA are inconsistent [4, 5], the type of exercise may play a role as one study showed a reduction in depression with aerobic exercise but not with resistance exercise [6]. While exercise therapy is effective in the short-term, there is however strong evidence for no long-term effectiveness of exercise on pain and function [7] which reflects a lack of long-term adherence to exercise.

The following sections will summarize the literature relating to the effects of exercise at the common OA sites of the knee, hip and hand. Exercise for spinal OA is beyond the scope of this chapter given the non-specific nature of low back pain. A discussion of the practical issues of exercise prescription such as the mode of delivery, dosage and adherence will then be provided.

2.1. Exercise and Knee OA

Research into the role of exercise has primarily focused on its effects on symptoms. However, more recently at the knee there has been interest in whether exercise can also lower knee joint loads and slow disease progression. Given that there is currently no cure for OA, identification of disease-modifying interventions is an important goal.

2.1.1. Effects on Knee Pain and Function

Exercise has been consistently shown to reduce knee pain and improve function in knee OA (Table 1). A recent Cochrane Review identified 32 clinical trials investigating a variety of land-based therapeutic exercise programs [8]. Results of a meta-analysis showed mean treatment benefits for both knee pain (standardised mean difference 0.40, 95% CI 0.30 to 0.50) and physical function (SMD 0.37, 95% CI 0.25 to 0.49). Although the treatment effects can be considered small, they are nevertheless similar to those effects achieved from simple analgesia and non-steroidal anti-inflammatory drugs. A summary of the different types of exercise programs for knee OA will now be presented.

a. Muscle Strengthening

Patients with knee OA typically exhibit reductions in muscle strength possibly as a consequence of reductions in physical activity and disuse or pain inhibition [9-12]. There is also evidence to suggest that inadequate strength may reduce the ability to sufficiently absorb load during dynamic activities [13] and therefore play a role in the development and progression of knee OA [12, 14]. Consequently, many studies have examined the effects of muscle strengthening programs on clinical symptoms and physical functioning.

The quadriceps are the largest group of muscles crossing the knee joint and have the greatest potential to generate and absorb forces at the knee. Given the hypothesized role of the quadriceps in the pathogenesis of knee OA [12, 14, 15], and the fact that quadriceps weakness has been consistently related to reduced physical function [16, 17] as well as a greater likelihood of functional decline [15, 18], it is not surprising that the majority of strengthening studies have focused primarily – or entirely – on this muscle group. Despite subtle differences in factors such as the exercise type, equipment used, and the intervention duration, intervention studies have shown consistent improvements in isokinetic and isometric knee extension strength after training as well as reductions in pain and physical disability. Recent meta-analyses and systematic reviews [8, 19] confirm these findings. While quadriceps strengthening exercises may be performed in a variety of modes including isometric, isotonic, isokinetic, concentric and eccentric as well as non-weight bearing or weight bearing, these reviews indicate that no particular method of strength training is superior to another [8, 19]. Thus, clinicians can prescribe the type of exercise that best suits the individual patient.

Although not well studied, it is possible that local mechanical factors influence the response to exercise. A recent Randomized Controlled Trial (RCT) in 107 people with medial knee OA found that a 12 week quadriceps strengthening program led to a significant improvement in knee pain only in those with neutrally aligned knees and not in those with *varus* malalignment despite comparable strength increases in both groups [20]. Knee malalignment could alter the line of action of the quadriceps force and this could increase compression forces on localized areas of articular cartilage [21, 22], counteracting the positive benefits of strengthening on knee pain in this group. Whether individuals with malalignment may benefit more from functional exercises emphasizing neuromuscular control and coordination needs to be evaluated. However, the findings suggest that factors such as knee alignment may need to be considered when prescribing exercise.

Very little is known about the role that the hip musculature plays in the pathophysiology of knee OA. The hip abductors and adductors are known to control pelvic motion in the frontal plane during walking gait [23]. It is believed that a drop in the pelvis towards the swing limb that results from weak stance-limb hip musculature (in particular, the hip abductors), can shift knee joint loading more medially and increase the risk of medial tibiofemoral OA development and/or progression. Chang *et al.* [21] conducted a longitudinal cohort study on 57 patients (103 knees) with mild to moderate radiographic knee OA. They found that those knees (n=86) that did not exhibit radiographic disease progression after 18 months had higher ipsilateral *internal* hip abduction moments (which they attributed to greater hip abductor strength) during gait than knees that showed signs of disease progression (n=17). Mundermann *et al.* [24] reported higher internal hip abduction moments during gait in individuals with mild to moderate knee OA compared to those with severe OA, further suggesting a protective effect of hip abduction strength against knee OA progression. These studies, in addition to recent findings of significant hip strength weaknesses in those with knee OA compared to those without [25] highlight the potential need for hip musculature strengthening in this patient population.

Table 1: Summary of trials (2004 and later) evaluating exercise for the improvement of pain and function for those with knee osteoarthritis.

References	Design	Population	Intervention	Follow-up	Outcomes measured	Results
Messier *et al.* (2004) [26]	RCT	158 obese individuals with knee OA	Exercise group received 48 class-based sessions (3 per week x 16 weeks) focusing on strengthening and aerobic walking. Follow-up home program that was monitored by telephone.	Baseline, 6 months, 18 months	- WOMAC pain - WOMAC function	- no significant improvement in function at any time point in the exercise only group (n=76) compared to the "healthy lifestyle education" group (n=78) - no significant improvement in pain in exercise only group
Keefe *et al.* (2004) [27]	RCT	34 individuals with knee OA	Exercise only group received 3 supervised exercise sessions (strength training, aerobic training, ROM training) per week over the 12-week intervention.	Baseline and post-treatment (12 weeks)	- AIMS pain	- no significant improvement in those who received exercise only compared to control group
Hughes *et al.* (2004) [28]	RCT	150 individuals with hip and knee OA (*proportions unknown)	Exercise group received 24 class-based sessions (muscle strengthening, aerobic conditioning, education) over the 8-week intervention.	Baseline, post-treatment (8 weeks), 6 months	- WOMAC pain - WOMAC function	- significant pain improvements only at 6 months - no significant improvement in function
Thorstensson *et al.* (2005) [29]	RCT	61 individuals with knee OA	Exercise group received 12 clinic-based sessions (2 per week x 6 weeks) of intensive muscle strengthening.	Baseline and post-treatment (6 weeks)	- KOOS pain - KOOS ADL	- no significant differences between those who did and did not receive the intervention

Bennell *et al.* (2005) [30]	RCT	140 individuals with knee OA	Exercise group received individual, comprehensive physiotherapy treatment (8 sessions over 12 weeks) that included massage, taping, and muscle strengthening.	Baseline and post-treatment (12 weeks)	- VAS pain - WOMAC function	- no significant differences between those who received the active and placebo treatments for both pain and function
Huang *et al.* (2005) [31]	RCT	140 individuals with bilateral knee OA	Exercise group received 24 individual sessions (3 per week x 8 weeks) of isokinetic muscle strengthening and ROM exercises	Baseline, post-treatment (8 weeks), 1 year	- VAS pain - Lequesne function	- significant improvements in pain and function in all groups (n=105) that received any exercise treatment - significant improvements maintained at follow-up compared to no treatment control group
Hay *et al.* (2006) [32]	RCT	325 individuals with knee pain	Exercise group received a pragmatic physiotherapy program combining coping strategies with an individualised exercise program (3-6 sessions over 10 weeks)	Baseline, post-intervention (3 months), 6 months, 12 months	- WOMAC pain - WOMAC function	- significant improvements in pain and function immediately following intervention compared to no treatment - between-group differences were no longer present by 6 months
Mikesky *et al.* (2006) [33]	RCT	221 community volunteers	Exercise group received 45 clinic sessions (in first 12 months) of isokinetic muscle strengthening. Participants then received a home strengthening program for the next 18 months.	Baseline, post-intervention (30 months)	- WOMAC pain - WOMAC function	- strength training group showed no overall improvements with pain compared to ROM group - trend towards better function in the strength training group * Note that both groups (strength and ROM) contained individuals without pain and/or clinical diagnosis of knee OA
Song *et al.* (2007) [34]	RCT	72 women with OA	Sun-style Tai Chi exercise - 3 times a week for first two weeks, and then once a week for 10 weeks.	Baseline, post intervention (12 weeks)	- WOMAC - Motivation for and health behaviours	- reductions in perceived arthritic symptoms and improved perception of health benefits to perform better health behaviours * Note large drop out rate of 41%
Brismee *et al.* (2007) [35]	RCT	41 individuals with knee OA	Tai chi programme - 6 weeks of group tai chi sessions, 40 min/session, 3 times a week, followed by another 6 weeks (weeks 7 -12) of home-based tai chi training.	Baseline then every 3 weeks until 18 weeks	- VAS pain - WOMAC function - WOMAC stiffness	-improvements in knee pain, physical function and stiffness compared to baseline in Tai Chi group but no significant change in attention control group -tai chi group had better pain and function than the attention control group at weeks 9 and 12. -All improvements disappeared after detraining.

Lim *et al.* (2008) [20]	RCT	107 individuals with knee OA, stratified by alignment	Exercise group received a 12-week, partially supervised targeted quadriceps strengthening program (7 consultations with physiotherapist)	Baseline, post-intervention (12 weeks)	- WOMAC pain - WOMAC function	- no significant improvement in function in either alignment group - significant improvement in pain only in those with more neutrally aligned lower limbs
Doi *et al.* (2008) [36]	RCT	121 individuals with knee OA	Exercise group received an 8 week partially supervised, home-based targeted quadriceps strengthening program	Baseline, post-intervention (8 weeks)	- WOMAC pain - VAS pain - SF-36 pain	- significant improvements in all pain measures after the intervention, though not statistically different than group who received NSAID therapy
Aglamis *et al.* (2008) [37]	RCT	34 individuals with knee OA	Exercise group received a 12-week combined program emphasizing lower limb functional strengthening and aerobic conditioning	Baseline, 6 weeks, post-intervention (12 weeks)	- VAS pain - SF-36 function - SF-36 pain	- significant improvements in all outcomes by 6 weeks, which was maintained until end of intervention
Jan *et al.* (2009) [38]	RCT	106 individuals with knee OA	Participants in the 2 exercise groups received either weight bearing or non-weight bearing resistance exercises for 8 weeks	Baseline, post-treatment (8 weeks)	- WOMAC function	- significant improvement in both groups compared to control, though no differences between weight bearing and non-weight bearing groups
Wang *et al.* (2009) [39]	RCT	40 individuals with knee OA	60 minutes of Tai Chi (10 modified forms from classic Yang style) twice weekly for 12 weeks.	Baseline, post-treatment (12 weeks), 24 weeks, 48 weeks	- WOMAC pain - WOMAC function - Global assessment - Timed chair stand - Depression index - Self efficacy - Quality of life	- compared with attention control group (wellness education and stretching), the Tai Chi group had significant improvements in all measures
Jenkinson *et al.* (2009) [40]	RCT	389 individuals aged > 45 with BMI ≥ 28 and self reported knee pain	Dietary intervention plus quadriceps strengthening exercises; dietary intervention alone; quadriceps strengthening exercises alone; advice leaflet only (control group)	Baseline, 6, 12 & 24 months	- WOMAC pain - WOMAC function - WOMAC stiffness - SF-36 - Hospital anxiety and depression scale	- significant reduction in knee pain and function in exercise groups compared with non-exercise groups at 24 months with moderate effect size.

RCT=randomised controlled trial; VAS=visual analogue scale; WOMAC=Western Ontario and McMaster Osteoarthritis Index, a disease-specific measure of pain, function and stiffness; SF-36=short form 36 measuring health-related quality of life; KOOS=Knee Injury and Osteoarthritis Outcome Score, a joint-specific self-report questionnaire assessing pain, symptoms, function, and activity participation; AIMS=Arthritis Impact Measurement Scale, a disease-specific self-report measure of the impact of arthritis on the patient; ROM=range of motion.

We have recently conducted the first RCT investigating the effects of targeted hip abductor and adductor strengthening in this patient population [41]. In this study, 89 patients with knee OA were randomized to either a 12-week, partially supervised hip strengthening program or usual care. Those in the exercise group exhibited significant increases in isometric abduction and adduction strength and improvements in self-reported pain and physical function. Results of this study indicate that improvements in knee OA symptoms can be achieved without targeting knee musculature, thereby providing an alternative treatment option for patients for whom traditional knee muscle strengthening exercises are too painful or difficult.

b. Aerobic Exercise

Aerobic exercise involves exercising for prolonged periods of time at an elevated intensity (approximately 60-80% of maximum heart rate). Common activities include swimming, walking, and cycling and all have been found to be effective in reducing symptoms of knee OA (Table 1). Structured walking programs have received particular interest in the treatment of knee OA given the familiarity, minimal need for equipment, and importance in activities of daily living. When compared to control groups, walking programs have been shown to reduce knee joint pain [42-44], improve physical functioning during activities such as stair climbing [45], increase aerobic capacity [46] and physical endurance [47, 48], and improve gait characteristics [48]. Additionally, Sharma *et al.* [18] found that the amount of aerobic exercise per week was predictive of long-term physical function (WOMAC physical function and time required for 5 chair stands) in a 3-year longitudinal cohort study of 236 individuals with knee OA.

Aerobic exercise also has the potential to reduce body mass – a well-known risk factor for knee OA development and progression [49-52]. Given the strong associations among body mass, knee joint loading, and articular cartilage degeneration, exercise programs that promote weight loss through aerobic activity appear warranted. Indeed, many clinicians advocate the use of some form of aerobic activity for individuals with knee OA, particularly those who are obese, and weight loss consistently appears in clinical guidelines for the treatment of knee OA [53].

c. Neuromuscular Retraining Programs

Many authors advocate the use of exercises emphasizing motor control strategies for individuals with knee OA given the combination of sensory and motor dysfunction in this patient population that contribute to the physical impairments commonly observed [54]. There is evidence showing that individuals with knee OA exhibit altered neuromuscular control strategies during tasks such as force targeting [55], walking [56, 57], and stair ascent/descent [56] compared to those without joint disease. Furthermore, a recent longitudinal study showed that poorer proprioceptive acuity was associated with slightly greater worsening of pain and physical function compared with those with the best proprioceptive acuity, whose pain and physical function score deteriorated less [58].

It is suggested that programs focusing on techniques to improve balance and coordination may be beneficial to improve skills required for activities of daily living. Indeed, Hurley [59] argues that maximizing strength gains are of little value if the individual lacks the neuromuscular control to perform functional activities. Instead, he suggests that the effects of exercise can be optimized by combining strength and endurance exercises with coordination and functional performance training and/or patient education.

Despite the rationale, there is limited research into the efficacy of exercise programs aiming to enhance neuromuscular control and balance/co-ordination in knee OA. In a case study, a structured agility and perturbation training program modified from that used for younger patients with anterior cruciate ligament insufficiency reduced symptoms of instability in an older woman with knee OA [60]. The program included activities such as side stepping, braiding, front and back cross over steps, shuttle walking, obstacle course and perturbations applied by a therapist while the patient tried to balance on various surfaces. One non-randomised study reported significant improvements in proprioception following a multi-faceted exercise program [61], while another randomised study demonstrated that the addition of kinesthesia and balance exercises to a strengthening programme did not offer any additional improvement in proprioceptive acuity than a strengthening programme alone [62]. Use of a computerized proprioception facilitation exercise was equally as effective as closed kinetic chain exercise in improving proprioception and symptoms compared with a no-exercise control group [63]. Another strategy may be to train patients to activate appropriate selective muscles through specific exercises [64] and using real-time biofeedback and motor control relearning. In this, the movement is broken down into smaller components and the person is made aware of the muscle activity required. Repetition and feedback are key components. Whether these techniques are effective has not been formally tested.

d. Tai Chi

Tai Chi is a popular form of exercise that involves slow controlled movement, relaxation and deep and regulated breathing techniques. It is thought to improve muscle strength, flexibility, balance and co-ordination. A systematic review located 12 clinical trials of tai chi for OA but only five were randomized [65]. It concluded that there is some encouraging evidence that tai chi may be effective for pain control and improving physical function but the evidence is not convincing and further research is needed. A more recent RCT investigated 60 minutes of tai chi (10 modified forms from classic Yang style) compared with attention control (wellness education and stretching) twice weekly for 12 weeks in 40 people with knee OA [39]. It found that tai chi reduces pain and improves physical function, self-efficacy, depression, and health-related quality of life for knee OA.

e. Combination Exercise Therapy

Although studies examining single exercise interventions (*e.g.* walking programs, quadriceps strengthening) provide valuable information on the effectiveness of these particular treatment methods, physiotherapists and other healthcare practitioners rarely advocate the use of a single intervention for the rehabilitation of most pathologies. This is especially relevant given that previous research has failed to find clear evidence to support one type of exercise over another [42, 46, 66, 67]. In contrast, the presumption that clinical outcome is maximized by the combination of different types of exercise or with other intervention strategies has been supported by much research.

Rogind *et al.* [68] and Suomi and Collier [69] conducted studies investigating changes in pain and function after the implementation of exercise programs that included strengthening, endurance, balance, range of motion, coordination, and general fitness. Both studies found favourable effects from these multifaceted exercise programs with significant reductions in pain and improvements in strength, walking speed, and self-reported physical function.

Messier *et al.* [26] showed in a group of 316 overweight individuals with radiographic evidence of knee OA that pain, function, and mobility were improved significantly greater after 18 months in the group of participants receiving dietary advice combined with aerobic and resistance exercise components than either intervention given in isolation. Additionally, those who received the exercise plus dietary advice lost more weight (5.7%) than those who received only dietary advice (4.9%) or exercise (3.7%), and significantly more than those who received healthy lifestyle education (1.2%). These results suggest that anatomical factors associated with knee OA (*i.e.* body mass) and clinical measures of symptoms and function can both be optimized with the combination of effective therapies.

Along with exercise, another core treatment component recommended by clinical guidelines is self-management interventions. Consistent with a biopsychosocial approach to the management of chronic conditions such as OA, self-management interventions can challenge inappropriate health beliefs and help people cope with their condition and adopt healthy lifestyles and behaviours [70]. While exercise and self-management interventions are generally delivered separately, there has been interest in examining whether there are additional benefits if rehabilitation programs integrate the two. A number of integrated programs have been reported in the literature varying widely in terms of their duration, delivery format and content of the individual components [70, 71]. In general, the results have shown that the integrated rehabilitation programs improve pain and function but with small and unimpressive benefits over and above exercise or self-management alone. Furthermore, some of the programs were long, complex, burdensome and expensive which would detract from widescale clinical implementation. More recently, programs have been devised that appear to be more acceptable [72, 73]. For example, a community-based integrated rehabilitation programme that was delivered in a group setting for people with chronic knee pain (ESCAPE-knee pain) was as effective in producing sustained physical and psychosocial benefits as usual outpatient physiotherapy but importantly the integrated program cost less and was more cost-effective [74].

2.1.2. Effects on Joint Loading

Despite consistently favourable clinical outcomes, until recently very little work has been conducted into the effects of exercise on mechanical factors associated with the disease at this joint. In this patient population, the external knee adduction moment is the most recognized measure of dynamic joint loading during walking and has been validated as an indirect measure of medial tibiofemoral joint load [75, 76]. Importantly, the knee adduction moment is associated with disease progression with higher adduction moment values increasing the likelihood of structural disease progression in the medial compartment [77]. Accordingly, the adduction moment has been the outcome measure of choice for studies examining the effects of exercise on knee joint load.

It is believed that by strengthening the lower limb musculature, more load can be absorbed by these muscles during walking, thereby unloading the diseased compartment, with a resultant decrease in the adduction moment. This could then potentially reduce the risk of disease progression. We are aware of only five studies that have measured the changes in adduction moment magnitudes following an exercise intervention. Thorstensson *et al.* [78] conducted a small 8-week pilot study on 13 individuals with knee OA that emphasized improving lower extremity muscle strength and neuromuscular coordination. King *et al.* [22] evaluated the effects of a 12-week high intensity knee extensor and flexor resistance training program on 14 patients with medial knee OA and *varus* malalignment. Lim *et al.* [20] conducted a randomized controlled trial with 107 individuals with knee OA where they were allocated either a 12-week supervised home-based quadriceps strengthening program or usual care. Our 12-week RCT targeted hip abductors and adductors muscle strengthening (n=89) [79] and finally a 6 month RCT compared high intensity lower limb resistance training with sham resistance training (n=54) [80] . Surprisingly none of these studies reported significant reductions in any measure of the knee adduction moment during walking following the intervention. More surprisingly was that most of these studies reported a small, but statistically non-significant, increase in the adduction moment during normal walking. The reason for these findings is unknown, especially in light of significant improvements in pain and function and typically no changes in walking speed, a factor that is associated with a higher adduction moment. Clearly more research in this area is needed given the importance of reducing joint loading in this patient population in addition to increasing the amount of physical activity.

2.1.3. Effects on Joint Structure

There is presently little evidence to suggest that stronger muscles can protect against OA progression in those with established disease. A longitudinal study on 79 participants with radiographic knee OA [81] found that the mean quadriceps strength of participants with progressive OA was about 9% lower than those with radiographically stable OA although this difference in strength between the groups was not statistically significant. In another longitudinal cohort study, Sharma and colleagues [18] showed that greater absolute quadriceps strength at baseline increased the risk of disease progression in people with malaligned knees but not in those with neutral alignment. Greater strength was also associated with an increased likelihood of progression in high-laxity knees. The authors suggested that the inability of malaligned knees to evenly distribute muscle forces could result in focal stress while the increase in muscle contraction to stabilize lax knees could lead to higher joint reaction forces. In contrast, using the more sensitive technique of magnetic resonance imaging to assess cartilage, Amin *et al.* [15] found no association between quadriceps strength and cartilage loss at the tibiofemoral joint with similar results seen in malaligned knees. However, greater quadriceps strength was protective against cartilage loss at the lateral compartment of the patellofemoral joint.

Only one clinical trial has specifically addressed the question of whether exercise influenced joint structure in people with knee OA. In this study, older adults with and without knee pain were randomly allocated to either a strength training or range of motion exercise group [33]. Exercise was initially supervised for 12 weeks and thereafter increasingly performed at home up until 30 months. Strength training was directed to both the upper and lower limbs but with an emphasis on quadriceps and hamstrings. Whilst participants in both exercise groups lost lower-extremity muscle strength over 30 months, the rate of loss was slower with strength training compared to range of motion exercises. In participants with established knee OA at baseline, the mean loss of joint space width measured by radiographs in the strengthening group was 37% less than that in the range of motion group, however this difference was not statistically significant. Semi-quantitative ratings of loss of joint space width revealed that joint space narrowing occurred less frequently in the strengthening group compared to range of motion exercise (18% vs 28%, p=0.094). Trends in data from this study suggest that lower limb strength training may have a role to play in slowing structural deterioration over time in established knee OA but further large-scale studies using more sensitive imaging techniques (such as MRI) and different forms of exercise are needed before conclusions can be drawn.

2.2. Exercise and Hip OA

There is much less attention on exercise for hip OA in the literature compared with knee OA and findings from studies involving patients with knee OA cannot necessarily be directly extrapolated to the hip given differences in biomechanics, impairments, rapidity of progression and risk factors. Therefore, while current international treatment guidelines recommend therapeutic exercise for people with symptomatic hip OA [2, 3], these recommendations are based on expert opinion only at this stage due to a dearth of research in this area.

Of the limited RCTs evaluating the effects of land-based exercise for hip OA (Table **2**), only one study exclusively recruited people with hip OA [82]. The other studies included people with hip and/or knee OA. This means that the exercise programs in these studies were not specifically designed for hip OA and may not necessarily address the relevant hip impairments. Furthermore the results were not joint-specific and there were inadequate numbers with hip OA to allow conclusions to be drawn for the hip joint. There is variation between the studies particularly with regards to the type, dosage, mode of delivery and duration of the exercise program (Table **2**). One program involved Tai Chi [83], whereas the others all included some form of lower limb strengthening. Aerobic land-based exercise such as walking has not been investigated. Home-based exercise was the delivery mode in two studies [84, 85] while the rest generally included exercise under the supervision of a physical therapist. The duration of the intervention ranged from 6-12 weeks except in one study where it was 24 weeks [85].

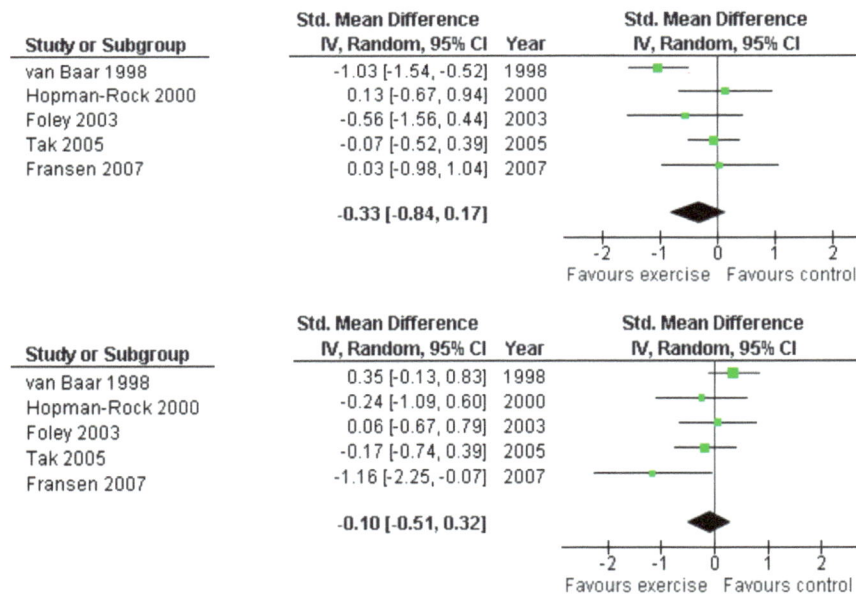

Study or Subgroup	Std. Mean Difference IV, Random, 95% CI	Year
van Baar 1998	-1.03 [-1.54, -0.52]	1998
Hopman-Rock 2000	0.13 [-0.67, 0.94]	2000
Foley 2003	-0.56 [-1.56, 0.44]	2003
Tak 2005	-0.07 [-0.52, 0.39]	2005
Fransen 2007	0.03 [-0.98, 1.04]	2007
	-0.33 [-0.84, 0.17]	

Favours exercise   Favours control

Study or Subgroup	Std. Mean Difference IV, Random, 95% CI	Year
van Baar 1998	0.35 [-0.13, 0.83]	1998
Hopman-Rock 2000	-0.24 [-1.09, 0.60]	2000
Foley 2003	0.06 [-0.67, 0.79]	2003
Tak 2005	-0.17 [-0.74, 0.39]	2005
Fransen 2007	-1.16 [-2.25, -0.07]	2007
	-0.10 [-0.51, 0.32]	

Favours exercise   Favours control

Figure 1: Forest plot for studies evaluating the effect of land-based exercise on change in (a) pain and (b) physical function in hip OA with permission [86].

In a recent Cochrane review of land-based exercise for hip OA, combining the results of five clinical trials demonstrated a small treatment effect for pain (Fig. **1a**), but no benefit in terms of improved self-reported physical function (Fig. **1b**) [86]. The authors concluded that the limited number and small sample size of the trials restricts the confidence that can be attributed to these results and that further clinical trials with larger sample sizes and exercise programs specifically designed for people with symptomatic hip OA need to be conducted. Similar conclusions were reached by the authors of another recent systematic review where it was stated that there was insufficient evidence to suggest that exercise therapy alone can be an effective short-term management approach for reducing pain levels, function, and quality of life [87]. Conversely, the results of another recent meta-analysis were more favourable in terms of the benefits of exercise for pain relief in hip OA but studies using water-based programs were also included in this meta-analysis [88]. The review concluded that therapeutic exercise, especially with specialized hand-on exercise training and an element of strengthening, is an efficacious treatment for hip OA [88].

2.3. Exercise and Hand OA

A Task Force of the EULAR standing committee for international clinical studies including therapeutics (ESCISIT) recommends that the optimal management of hand OA includes rehabilitative interventions, such as joint protection, education, exercise, splints, and heat, however, the level of evidence supporting this recommendation was reported as being mainly at the level of 'expert opinion' because of limited research [89].

Table 2: Summary of randomised controlled trials evaluating land-based exercise for the management of hip osteoarthritis.

References	Design	Population	Intervention	Follow-up	Outcomes measured	Results
Van Baar *et al.* (1998) [90]	RCT	Hip OA (n=71) and knee OA (n=119) and both (n=10)	1) 12 weeks of 1-3x/wk, 30 minute sessions comprising exercises for muscle strength, mobility, movement, locomotion, and coordination 2) usual care by the general practitioners	Baseline and 12 weeks	- VAS pain - Observed disability - Medication use	Exercise therapy was associated with a reduction of pain in the past week and observed disability. Effect sizes were medium (0.58) and small (0.28), respectively.
Hopman-Rock and Westhoff (2000) [84]	RCT	Hip OA and knee OA (n=120 in total; breakdown for each site not given)	1) 6 weeks of home-based 1x/wk, 60 minute session comprising strengthening exercises for hip/knee (+ health education program) 2) no treatment	Baseline, 6 weeks and 6 months	- Pain - Quality of life - Muscle strength - Range of motion - Activity restrictions - Body mass index (BMI) - Knowledge of OA and self efficacy - Health care utilisation	Benefits were found for pain, quality of life, quads strength, knowledge, self-efficacy, BMI, physically active lifestyle, and visits to the physical therapist. Most effects were moderate at posttest assessment and smaller at followup. No effects were found for range of motion and functional tasks.
Foley *et al.* (2003) [91]	RCT	Hip OA (n=35) and knee OA (n=83)	1) 6 weeks of 3x/wk, 30 minute sessions of strengthening exercises 2) Fortnightly telephone calls	Baseline and 6 weeks	- WOMAC - Quadriceps strength - 6 minute walk test - Adelaide Activities Profile - SF-12 - Arthritis Self Efficacy Scale	Gym program significantly improved quads strength, walking speed and self efficacy compared with the control group but did not reduce pain

Ravaud *et al.* (2004) [85]	Cluster RCT	Hip OA (n=741) and knee OA (n=2216)	1) 24 weeks of a home-based exercise program to improve muscle strength and range of motion daily at least 4x/wk 2) Usual care	Baseline and 24 weeks	- VAS pain - WOMAC	Home exercise did not lead to significantly greater benefits than usual care after 6 months in patients with OA concurrently receiving nonsteroidal anti-inflammatory drugs
Tak *et al.* (2005) [82]	RCT	109 people with hip OA	1) 8 weeks of 1x/wk, 60 minute session comprising strengthening exercises, treadmill 2) Usual care	Baseline, 8 weeks and 12 weeks	- VAS pain - Harris Hip Score - Sickness Impact Profile - Groningen Activity Restriction Scale - Timed functional tests - Quality of life (QOL)	Exercise had a positive effect on pain (moderate effect at post-test and small effect at followup), hip function (small effect at post-test), self-reported disability (small effect at followup), and the timed Up & Go test (small effect at followup). It did not affect QOL, other measures of observed disability, or BMI.
Fransen *et al.* (2007) [83]	RCT	Hip OA (n=20) and knee OA (n=77)	1) 12 weeks of 2x/wk (24 x 1 hour sessions) comprising class-based Sun style Tai Chi 2) Wait list control	Baseline, 12 weeks and 24 weeks	- WOMAC - General health status SF-12 - Depression, Anxiety and Stress Scale DASS21 - Patient global rating of change - Timed functional tests	Tai Chi resulted in significant improvements in function compared with controls with a moderate effect size (0.63) but no effect on pain. Benefits were sustained at follow-up

RCT=randomised controlled trial; VAS=visual analogue scale; WOMAC=Western Ontario and McMaster Osteoarthritis Index, a disease-specific measure of pain, function and stiffness; SF-36=short form 36 measuring health-related quality of life.

There are three small RCTs that have evaluated exercise in people with OA of the hand affecting the carpometacarpal and/or interphalangeal joints (Table 3). Two of the studies employed daily home exercises [92, 93] while the other was a therapist-supervised program performed three times per week [94]. One of the exercise programs comprised purely range of motion exercises as it was felt that applying resistance to exercises may be detrimental [93], one comprised only strengthening exercises [94] and the other included a combination of strengthening and range of motion exercises [92] (Table 4). The duration of the interventions ranged from 6 weeks to 4 months. One study also utilised a sham treatment of daily application of hand cream in the comparison group [92].

In general all studies showed improvements in grip strength with exercise but none of the studies showed benefits with respect to pain levels. The effects of exercise on hand function were inconsistent. One of the limitations includes the small sample sizes with most studies likely to be underpowered to detect clinically relevant improvements. Further research is therefore required to determine the most appropriate content and dosage of exercise programs for the treatment of hand OA.

3. PRACTICAL EXERCISE PRESCRIPTION

This section will cover the practical issues in relation to exercise prescription including the mode of delivery, dosage and adherence to exercise. It is important to note however that the research in this area relates mainly to knee OA and as such the findings may not necessarily translate to exercise for OA at other sites. A summary of exercise recommendations for clinical practice from the MOVE consensus [3] are found in Table 5.

3.1. Mode of delivery

Exercise may be delivered *via* individual treatments, supervised group classes or performed at home. Advantages of group-based exercise programs include the social aspects of group therapy and the ability to minimize resources and cost. Disadvantages include greater difficulty in tailoring exercise to individual patients and the need for patients to attend a specific location at a set time. Home exercise entails little financial outlay and provides the patient with greater flexibility regarding timing of the exercise session. However, there is a lack of supervision and often a lack of suitable equipment.

It appears that all three modes of exercise delivery are effective in reducing symptoms [8]. However, therapist contact may improve outcomes. McCarthy *et al.* [95] studied the effects of supplementing a home-based exercise program with physiotherapist-supervised exercise program for eight weeks. At the 12-month follow-up assessment, patients who received the home-based program supplemented with the 8-week group exercise class exhibited significant improvements in locomotor function and walking pain. The number of directly supervised exercise sessions can also influence treatment effect sizes. In a recent meta-analysis, studies evaluating exercise programs with less than 12 direct supervision occasions demonstrated small treatment effects whereas those with more than 12 direct supervision occasions demonstrated moderate treatment effects [8, 19].

One mode of exercise delivery that has been shown to be ineffective is a "minimalist" approach whereby patients are simply given a pamphlet or audiovisual material outlining a standardized exercise program. In a large study, this exercise approach delivered by rheumatologists yielded similar clinical outcomes to usual care after 6 months [85]. Numerous factors likely contributed to the ineffectiveness of exercise in this study. Patients were poorly compliant and an unsupervised standardized exercise program and dosage was used which may have been ineffective for such a heterogeneous patient group. Whilst a videotape demonstration of the exercises was provided, it would appear that technology is no substitute for personal demonstration. As a result, it is possible that many patients were performing the exercises incorrectly, further reducing their effectiveness.

It is suggested then that optimal improvements in symptoms and function may be achieved through the use of both individualized and group exercise treatment sessions followed by a home program. This may also alleviate some of the financial burdens associated with patient care in this population.

3.2. Dosage

The frequency, duration and intensity of the exercise program may affect clinical outcomes but these have not been well studied in people with OA. Although a definitive dose-based response to exercise has been reported, there may be issues with maintaining high compliance in programs with long durations. Most exercise guidelines would suggest a physiological response can be attained with as little as three exercise sessions per week, and research into the effectiveness of exercise programs in individuals with knee OA have shown improvements after 8- or 12-week programs [3].

The optimal intensity of a strengthening program is unclear. High-intensity training (high resistance/load) might be expected to result in greater strength gains than low-intensity training but could potentially overload the joint and exacerbate symptoms such as pain, inflammation and swelling. A recent study compared the effects of 8 weeks of high- and low-intensity closed kinetic chain knee strengthening exercise performed thrice weekly in 102 people with knee OA [96]. High-intensity training was defined as 3 sets of 8 repetitions with an exercise weight set initially at 60% of one repetition maximum whilst low-intensity training was defined as 10 sets of 15 repetitions with an initial exercise weight of 10% of one repetition maximum. This ensured that both groups were performing a similar overall volume of mechanical work. The results showed that both strengthening programs were beneficial for pain, function, walking time and muscle strength. However, although not significantly different, the effect sizes were larger for high resistance strength training. From a practical perspective, the high-intensity program took 20 minutes less compliance.

The current consensus recommendations by the American College of Sports Medicine and the American Heart Association for exercise and physical activity levels for older adults provide a guide for people with OA to aim toward [97].

Table 3: Summary of clinical trials evaluating exercise for the management of hand osteoarthritis.

References	Design	Population	Intervention	Follow-up	Outcomes measured	Results
Stamm *et al.* (2002) [93]	RCT	40 patients with hand OA	1) Joint protection advice + daily home hand exercise program (7 range of motion exercises) for 3 months 2) One information session about hand OA + non slip matting for opening jars	Baseline and 3 months	- VAS general pain - Grip strength - VAS global hand function - Health assessment questionnaire	Grip strength improved by 25% in the joint protection and exercise group, but not in the control group. Global hand function improved in a significantly larger proportion of patients in the exercise group (65%) than the control group (20%). No difference in hand pain
Lefler *et al.* (2004) [94]	RCT	19 patients with hand OA	1) Strengthening exercises - therapist supervised 3x/wk approximately 10 minutes per session for 6 weeks 2) No treatment	Baseline and 6 weeks	- Pain on 0-6 scale - Grip and pinch strength - Finger range of motion with goniometer	There was no effect of exercise on pain levels or pinch strength but there was a greater improvement in grip strength and range of motion with exercise
Rogers *et al.* (2009) [92]	Randomised, cross-over	46 patients with hand OA	1) Daily home-based hand exercise program (9 range of motion and strengthening exercises) for 4 months 2) Sham hand cream	Baseline and 4 months	- Australian/Canadian osteoarthritis hand index (AUSCAN) - Grip, key pinch and 3-finger chuck pinch strength - Dexterity – hand pin placement test	Changes in AUSCAN sub-scales did not differ between exercise and sham treatments. No changes in dexterity were seen. Grip and pinch measures modestly improved after exercise but not sham

RCT=randomised controlled trial; VAS=visual analogue scale;

These recommend that resistance exercise is performed at least twice weekly, including progressive weight training of 8-10 exercises of the major muscle groups for 8-12 repetitions, performed at a moderate to vigorous intensity. For endurance exercise, it is recommended that individuals accumulate at least 30 minutes and up to 60 minutes per day of moderate intensity activities in bouts of at least 10 minutes each to total 150-300 minutes per week. Importantly, a recent study showed that around 70% of people with mild knee OA did not achieve recommended levels for moderate physical activity [98]. This highlights the need to incorporate strategies to increase general physical activity levels in people with OA.

4. ENHANCING UPTAKE OF EXERCISE AND PATIENT ADHERENCE

The challenge remains to increase the proportion of patients with OA exercising. Whilst there are many barriers to the uptake of exercise in the OA population, there are three of particular importance; i) recommendation of exercise to patients by medical practitioners and appropriate referral to exercise professionals; ii) evidence-based use of exercise therapy by therapists and; iii) adherence by patients to prescribed exercise programs.

Exercise is under-utilized by medical practitioners as a treatment strategy for OA [99]. In a survey of 3000 French general practitioners, less than 15% reported that they would prescribe exercise for knee OA as a first line therapeutic approach. A survey of patients with OA in Canada revealed that only one-third had been advised to use exercise for their condition [100], however 73% reported that they had tried exercise in the past. Given the large number of patients who chose to try exercise independently, it is possible that many failed to consult a professional regarding the most appropriate exercise to commence.

It is important to ensure that therapists are prescribing appropriate exercise and facilitating behavioural change in patients with OA. A recent study reported on the results of a UK survey of over 1,100 physical therapists' use of therapeutic exercise for OA [101]. It found that therapists mostly used local exercises such as strengthening and range of motion exercises over more general exercise or a combination of exercise types that has been recommended. It also showed that the exercise was delivered over relatively few treatment sessions with limited supervision and monitoring following discharge all of which could potentially reduce the exercise benefits. The survey plus semi-structured interviews were used together to explore therapists' beliefs and attitudes regarding exercise and OA [102]. This study revealed that many therapists largely worked under a biomedical framework whereby they viewed OA as a progressive 'wear and tear' disease. This may have contributed to their uncertainty about the benefits and safety of exercise for OA and their adoption of a pain-contingent approach to exercise prescription. The study also showed that therapists tended to adopt a paternalistic approach that emphasized the patient's responsibility in long-term adherence to exercise rather than viewing it as a shared responsibility. Thus, strategies need to be implemented that support therapists to provide clinical care in line with exercise recommendations for OA.

Patient adherence to exercise is often good during the first few months of commencing an exercise program but declines rapidly over time. Patient adherence is a key factor in determining outcome from exercise therapy in patients with knee OA [103]. Many studies have reported significant differences in outcome response after an exercise intervention based on the number of completed sessions with those individuals exhibiting higher adherence to the program achieving more beneficial results [103].

Table 5: Summary of evidence-based recommendations for exercise in knee and hip OA [3].

Proposition
• Both strengthening and aerobic exercise can reduce pain and improve function and health status.
• There are few contraindications to prescription of strengthening or aerobic exercise.
• Prescription of both general (aerobic fitness training) and local (strengthening) exercises is an essential, core aspect of management.
• Exercise therapy should be individualized and patient-centred taking into account factors such as age, co-morbidity and overall mobility.
• To be effective, exercise programmes should include advice and education to promote a positive lifestyle change with an increase in physical activity.
• Group exercise and home exercise are equally effective and patient preference should be considered.
• Adherence is the principle predictor of long-term outcome from exercise.
• Strategies to improve and maintain adherence should be adopted.
• Effectiveness of exercise is independent of presence or severity of x-ray findings.
• Improvements in muscle strength and proprioception gained from exercise programmes may reduce the progression of OA.

Although not well studied, a complex array of possible factors can contribute to adherence rates for exercise programs in individuals with OA. These are summarised in Fig. **2** and can be divided into different categories including psychological factors, intervention-related factors, and disease- and illness-related factors [104]. Adherence is improved when patients receive attention from health professionals rather than a primarily home-based exercise program [105]. Psychosocial attributes of the individual also influence adherence. Better adherence to therapy has been found to be related to the perception of more severe knee symptoms, belief in the effectiveness of the intervention, and understanding of the pathogenesis of knee OA (those who are less compliant tend to believe that OA is part of the natural ageing process or that it is simply a "wear and tear" disease) [106]. Self-efficacy, or one's belief in their own ability to perform tasks, is also associated with higher compliance and better outcome [104].

Many strategies have been suggested to improve patient adherence when prescribing exercise interventions for those with knee OA. Catering the exercise program to the unique requirements of the patient as well as ensuring availability of resources can be effective in maximizing compliance. Other methods suggested to improve compliance include: monitoring *via* telephone contact [107] or self-reported diary [108-110], graphic feedback [108], or lifestyle retraining [111]. While monitoring from a health care professional is the preferred method of contact, patients can rely on their own social support network when an appropriate health care professional is unavailable [110]. Additionally, self-monitoring *via* positive feedback loops based on level of physical function and attainment of goals may be useful for some patients. Potential strategies to facilitate long-term adherence to exercise are show in Table **6**.

Table 6: Suggestions to facilitate long-term adherence to exercise in OA [103, 104].

- Initiate exercise under expert instruction in the context of a clinical setting.
- Adjust exercise dosage accordingly if patient has difficulty.
- Take care to minimise undue negative affect, and self-efficacy related to exercise and outcome expectations of exercise should be maximized.
- Patient education - basic and accurate information about the disease and the benefits of exercise for OA of all severities.
- Long-term monitoring review by a health care professional by phone or mail.
- Regular follow-up or booster sessions.
- Inclusion of spouse/family in exercise program.
- Support from family and friends.
- Psychological support.
- Self-monitoring by means of diary, pedometer.

5. MANUAL THERAPY

Manual therapy is practiced by a range of health care professionals such as physical therapists, chiropractors, osteopaths, physiatrists and massage therapists. While manual therapy may be defined differently according to each profession, it generally refers to skilled hands-on techniques where accurately determined and specifically directed manual force is applied to the body. The purported aims of manual therapy include reducing pain; increasing range of motion and mobility; reducing soft tissue inflammation; increasing circulation; improving soft tissue repair; inducing relaxation; facilitating movement; and improving function.

Manual therapy comprises a number of techniques, the most common being manipulation and mobilisation. Manipulation techniques are defined as forceful small-amplitude, high-velocity movements of a joint often applied at end range [112]. Mobilisation techniques are repetitive passive movement of low velocity and varying amplitudes applied at different points throughout range [112]. Other techniques include soft tissue mobilisation and stretching and myofascial techniques. Massage may also be considered by some to be a form of manual therapy and thus will be reviewed in this section.

Manual therapy is commonly used in clinical practice for OA with surveys revealing that 96% of Irish physical therapists [113] and 64% of UK therapists [114] include it in their management of patients with hip and knee OA respectively. Despite its common usage, there is limited research on the effects of manual therapy for the treatment of OA and few studies have evaluated it in isolation from other interventions such as exercise.

One repeated-measures study examined the immediate effects of accessory knee joint mobilisation in 38 people with knee OA [115] (Table **7**). Large-amplitude oscillatory anterior-posterior glides of the knee joint performed for 9-minutes were compared with manual contact and no-contact interventions applied in random order in different test sessions separated by at least 2 days. Results showed that the mobilizations produced local and widespread hypoalgesia as indicated by increases in pressure pain thresholds. This study supports the potential pain-relieving benefits of manual therapy.

To date only two randomised controlled trials have evaluated the specific effects of manual therapy, other than massage, for the management of OA [116] (Table **7**). One high quality study compared a 5 week manual therapy program comprising mobilisation and manipulation of the hip joint with a therapist-supervised exercise program in 109 patients with hip OA [116]. Both groups showed improvement but the success rate in the manual therapy group (81%) was significantly better than that in the exercise group (50%). Benefits in favour of manual therapy were maintained at a 29-week follow-up. There was no differential response to manual therapy in specific subgroups of hip OA patients defined on the basis of baseline levels of hip function, pain and range of motion. However, patients with mild or moderate radiological grading of OA had better range of motion outcomes with manual therapy than those with severe radiological OA [117]. This study provides strong support for the role of manual therapy in the management of hip OA.

The other study to specifically evaluate manual therapy compared a chiropractic protocol to a control intervention comprising palmar contact to the knee without the application of force followed by interferential set at zero in 43 patients with knee OA [118] (Table 7). The protocol consisted of a myofascial mobilization procedure and an impact thrust procedure specific to the patellofemoral joint. Following the two week intervention there was a significant reduction in knee pain in the manual therapy group with no change in the control group. However, the study had a number of methodological issues including lack of blinding of participants and assessor, and lack of baseline comparability between groups weakening the strength of the findings. Several large clinical trials specifically evaluating manual therapy in patients with hip and knee OA are currently underway that will provide further evidence on completion [119, 120].

In clinical practice, manual therapy is generally not applied in isolation to treat OA but is combined with other interventions such as exercise. While high quality studies have investigated multimodal programs including manual therapy, obviously the effects specifically attributed to manual therapy cannot be ascertained from these [121, 122]. One randomised controlled trial compared a clinically-based program comprising individualised manual therapy, supervised exercise and home exercises with a home exercise program over 4 weeks in 134 people with knee OA [121]. The manual therapy techniques included muscle stretches and soft tissue and joint mobilisation. Results showed that the clinic treatment group improved to a significantly greater extent than the home exercise group.

Table 7: Summary of trials evaluating manual therapy techniques including massage for the management of lower limb osteoarthritis.

References	Design	Population	Intervention	Follow-up	Outcomes measured	Results
Hoeksma *et al.* (2004) [116]	RCT	109 patients with hip OA	All patients treated 2x/wk for 5 weeks (9 treatment sessions) 1) Manual therapy – muscle stretches and hip joint traction followed by traction manipulation 2) Exercise – strengthening, range of motion, stretches, walking, balance	Baseline, 5 weeks, 17 weeks, 29 weeks	- Self reported general improvement - SF-36 - Harris Hip Score - Hip range by goniometer - VAS main symptom - Time to walk 80 m	81% success rate in manual therapy group versus 50% in exercise group as well as greater improvements in pain, stiffness, hip function, range of motion and stiffness with manual therapy. Effects of manual therapy maintained after 29 weeks
Perlman *et al.* (2006) [123]	RCT	68 patients with knee OA	1) Swedish massage full body – 60 min sessions 2x/wk in weeks 1-4 and 1 x/wk in weeks 5-8 2) Usual care followed by delayed intervention	Baseline, 8 weeks and 16 weeks	- WOMAC - VAS pain - Time to walk 15 m - Knee range by goniometer	Significant improvements in pain and function after the intervention that largely persisted at 16 weeks. Massage was well tolerated. Large effect sizes – 0.64 to 0.86

Moss *et al.* (2007) [115]	Within-subject design	38 patients with knee OA	Each participant received each 9 minute treatment in random order over 3 sessions 1) Mobilization – large-amplitude anterior-posterior glide of tibia on femur 2) Manual contact – therapist hand positioning but no movement 3) No contact control	Baseline and post treatment (in same session)	- Pressure pain threshold - VAS pain on walking - Timed 'up and go' test - WOMAC function	Manual therapy immediately increased pressure pain thresholds at painful and non-painful distal site and reduced 'up and go' times.
Field *et al.* (2007) [124]	RCT	22 patients with hand OA	1) Massage on wrist /hand × 1x/wk + daily home self-massage for 4 weeks 2) No treatment	Baseline and 4 weeks	- VAS pain anchored with 5 faces - Perceived grip strength	Significant benefits of massage on pain. No effect on grip strength
Pollard *et al.* (2008) [118]	RCT	43 patients with knee OA	Patients treated 3x/wk for 2 weeks 1) Manual therapy – myofascial mobilisation to patellofemoral joint and myofascial impulse thrust 2) Control – palmar contact to the knee and interferential set at zero	Baseline, 2 weeks	- VAS pain	Greater reduction in pain following myofascial treatment than control

RCT=randomised controlled trial; VAS=visual analogue scale; WOMAC=Western Ontario and McMaster Osteoarthritis Index, a disease-specific measure of pain, function and stiffness; SF-36=short form 36 measuring health-related quality of life.

Another randomised trial by the same investigators found that manual therapy applied to the knee as well as to the lumbar spine, hip, and ankle as required, and a standardized knee exercise program for 4 weeks led to clinically and statistically significant functional improvements at 4 and 8 weeks compared with placebo treatment [122].

Table 8: Manual therapy techniques for the hip as described in the studies by Hoeksma *et al.* (2004) [116] and MacDonald *et al.* (2006) [112].

Technique	Description	Dosage
Muscle stretching [116]	Performed in supine- iliopsoas, quads, tensor fascia latae, gracilis, sartorius, adductors	Each muscle group: 8-10 second stretch, 2 times each
Hip joint traction manipulation [116]	Performed in supine. Therapist's hands placed above ankle. Performed in 30° abduction. With each manipulation, the hip joint is placed in a more limited position with the final one being in the most limited position. Can be progressed into less abduction (not less than 15°) and internal rotation	Maximum of 5 manipulations - In between manipulations, active-assisted hip joint motions are performed for relaxation
Nonthrust long-axis oscillation mobilization/manipulation [112]	Performed in supine. Therapist's hands placed just above ankle. Gentle and progressive long-axis distraction oscillations	Progressive increase in intensity and moving into more hip abduction and more flexion

Nonthrust medial mobilization/manipulation [112]	Performed in sidelying to promote medial and inferior articular mobility of the femoral head in the acetabulum and to improve hip abduction and internal rotation	NS
Lateral nonthrust mobilization/manipulation with a belt [112]	Performed in supine with hip flexed 90°. Belt applied around upper thigh and therapist to achieve a combined lateral femoral glide with hip internal rotation	NS
Prone figure-four nonthrust mobilization/manipulation [112]	Performed in prone with knee slightly off table. Therapist hand placed over buttock to apply an anterior glide to the femoral head.	NS
2 therapist sidelying medial nonthrust mobilization/manipulation with distraction [112]	Performed in sidelying. One therapist applies distraction force with hands placed above ankle. The other therapist applies a medial and inferior translation of the femoral head	Generally an oscillatory glide at middle to end range

NS=not stated

Importantly, at 1 year, 20% of patients in the placebo group versus 5% of patients in the treatment group had undergone knee arthroplasty suggesting that manual therapy and exercise may delay or prevent the need for surgical intervention. Such a finding has considerable cost-implications.

Therapeutic massage has only been evaluated in two clinical trials in OA, one in people with knee OA [123] and one in people with hand OA [124] (Table **7**). The study in 68 people with knee OA compared an 8-weeks course of 60-minutes massage sessions once to twice weekly with usual care [123]. The therapists used standard Swedish full-body massage that included: (i) Petrissage – compression or manipulation of soft tissue between the fingers and thumb; (ii) Effleurage – gliding of hands over the skin and soft tissues; and (iii) Tapotement – percussion-based massage where hands strike soft tissue in a repetitive, rhythmic fashion. Results showed significant improvements in pain and function immediately after the treatment that generally persisted at short-term follow-up. Effect sizes were large ranging from 0.64 to 0.86. The other study investigated the effects of 4-weeks of massage as compared to no treatment in a small number of people with hand OA [124]. It found that the massage group had significantly greater reductions in pain than the no treatment group although the size of the difference may not be clinically meaningful (mean difference in pain on VAS = -1.18, 95% CI = -2.10 to -0.26). Furthermore, in both massage studies there was no control for the therapist contact time making it difficult to attribute any improvements to the specific effects of massage.

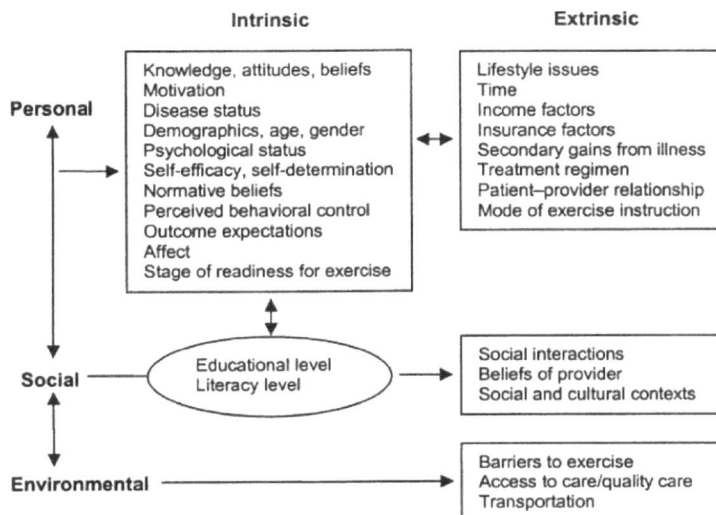

Figure 2: Potential factors influencing adherence to exercise programs by patients with osteoarthritis – reprinted with permission from Marks and Allegrante 2004 [104].

In summary, limited evidence suggests that manual therapy techniques may be beneficial in the management of large joint OA. Recently published UK clinical guidelines recommended manual therapy as an adjunctive treatment to core treatments of exercise and education in OA, particularly for hip OA [1]. The techniques used in the studies at the hip and knee are summarized in Tables **8** and **9** respectively. No studies have investigated the effects of manual therapy techniques, other than massage, for OA of the hand so the benefits for this patient group are largely unknown.

CONCLUDING REMARKS

Exercise is a core component of the management of people with OA. At this stage, there is no evidence to support the effectiveness of one type of exercise over another although a combination of strengthening and aerobic exercise is recommended. To maximize longer-term outcomes with exercise, strategies to promote adherence to exercise are needed. Manual therapy may be a useful adjunct to core treatment strategies for OA especially at the hip joint.

REFERENCES

[1] Conaghan PG, Dickson J, Grant RL. Care and management of osteoarthritis in adults: summary of NICE guidance. BMJ 2008; 336(7642): 502-3.

[2] Zhang W, Moskowitz RW, Nuki G, *et al.* OARSI recommendations for the management of hip and knee osteoarthritis, Part II: OARSI evidence-based, expert consensus guidelines. Osteoarthritis Cart 2008; 16(2): 137-62.

[3] Roddy E, Zhang W, Doherty M, *et al.* Evidence-based recommendations for the role of exercise in the management of osteoarthritis of the hip or knee- the MOVE consensus. Rheumatology 2005; 44(1): 67-73.

[4] Devos-Comby L, Cronan T, Roesch SC. Do exercise and self-management interventions benefit patients with osteoarthritis of the knee? A metaanalytic review. J Rheum 2006; 33(4): 744-56.

[5] Lange AK, Vanwanseele B, Fiatarone Singh MA. Strength training for treatment of osteoarthritis of the knee: a systematic review. Arthritis Rheum 2008; 59(10): 1488-94.

[6] Penninx BW, Rejeski WJ, Pandya J, Miller ME, Di Bari M, Applegate WB *et al.* Exercise and depressive symptoms: a comparison of aerobic and resistance exercise effects on emotional and physical function in older persons with high and low depressive symptomatology. J Gerontol B Psychol Sci Soc Sci 2002; 57(2): P124-32.

[7] Pisters MF, Veenhof C, van Meeteren NL, Ostelo RW, de Bakker DH, Schellevis FG *et al.* Long-term effectiveness of exercise therapy in patients with osteoarthritis of the hip or knee: a systematic review. Arthritis Rheum 2007; 57(7): 1245-53.

[8] Fransen M, McConnell S. Exercise for osteoarthritis of the knee. Cochrane Database of Systematic Reviews 2008; 4: 1-55.

[9] Hall KD, Hayes KW, Falconer J. Differential strength decline in patients with osteoarthritis of the knee: revision of a hypothesis. Arthritis Care Res 1993; 6(2): 89-96.

[10] Hassan BS, Mockett S, Doherty M. Static postural sway, proprioception, and maximal voluntary quadriceps contraction in patients with knee osteoarthritis and normal control subjects. Ann Rheum Dis 2001; 60(6): 612-8.

[11] Messier SP, Loeser RF, Hoover JL, Semble EL, Wise CM. Osteoarthritis of the knee: effects on gait, strength, and flexibility. Arch Phys Med Rehabil 1992; 73(1): 29-36.

[12] Slemenda C, Brandt KD, Heilman DK, Mazzuca S, Braunstein EM, Katz BP *et al.* Quadriceps weakness and osteoarthritis of the knee. Ann Intern Med 1997; 127: 97-104.

[13] Mikesky AE, Meyer A, Thompson KL. Relationship between quadriceps strength and rate of loading during gait in women. J Orthop Res 2000; 18: 171-5.

[14] Slemenda C, Heilman D, Brandt K, Katz B, Mazzuca SA, Braunstein E *et al.* Reduced quadriceps strength relative to body weight: a risk factor for knee osteoarthritis in women? Arthritis Rheum 1998; 41: 1951-9.

[15] Amin S, Baker K, Niu J, Clancy M, Goggins J, Guermazi A *et al.* Quadriceps strength and the risk of cartilage loss and symptom progression in knee osteoarthritis. Arthritis Rheum 2009; 60(1): 189-98.

[16] Maly MR, Costigan PA, Olney SJ. Determinants of self-report outcome measures in people with knee osteoarthritis. Arch Phys Med Rehabil 2006; 87(1): 96-104.

[17] van Dijk GM, Veenhof C, Lankhorst GJ, Dekker J. Limitations in activities in patients with osteoarthritis of the hip or knee: the relationship with body functions, comorbidity and cognitive functioning. Disabil Rehabil 2009; 31(20): 1685-91.

[18]   Sharma L, Cahue S, Song J, Hayes K, Pai Y, Dunlop D. Physical functioning over three years in knee osteoarthritis. Role of psychosocial, local mechanical, and neuromusculsr factors. Arthritis Rheum 2003; 48: 3359-70.

[19]   Pelland L, Brosseau L, Wells G, MacLeay L, Lambert J, Lamothe C *et al.* Efficacy of strengthening exercises for osteoarthritis (Part I): A meta-analysis. Phys Ther Rev 2004; 9:77-108.

[20]   Lim B, Hinman R, Wrigley T, Sharma L, Bennell K. Does knee malalignment mediate the effects of quadriceps strengthening on knee adduction moment, pain, and function in medial knee osteoarthritis? A randomized controlled trial. Arthritis Care Res 2008; 59: 943-51.

[21]   Chang A, Hayes K, Dunlop D, Song J, Hurwitz D, Cahue S *et al.* Hip abduction moment and protection against medial tibiofemoral osteoarthritis progression. Arthritis Rheum 2005; 52: 3515-9.

[22]   King L, Birmingham T, Kean C, Jones I, Bryant D, Giffin J. Resistance training for medial compartment knee osteoarthritis and malalignment. Med Sci Sports Ex 2008; 40: 1376-84.

[23]   Perry J. Gait analysis: Normal and pathologic function. Thorofare, NJ: Slack, Inc.; 1992.

[24]   Mundermann A, Dyrby C, Andriacchi T. Secondary gait changes in patients with medial compartment knee osteoarthritis: increased load at the ankle, knee, and hip during walking. Arthritis Rheum 2005; 52: 2835-44.

[25]   Hinman RS, Hunt MA, Creaby MW, Wrigley TV, McManus FJ, Bennell KL. Hip muscle weakness in individuals with medial knee osteoarthritis. Arthritis Care Res 2010;62(8):1190-3.

[26]   Messier S, Loeser R, Miller G, Morgan T, Rejeski W, Sevick M *et al.* Exercise and dietary weight loss in overweight and obese older adults with knee osteoarthritis. Arthritis Rheum 2004; 50(5): 1501-10.

[27]   Keefe F, Blumenthal J, Baucom D, Affleck G, Waugh R, Caldwell D *et al.* Effects of spouse-assisted coping skills training and exercise training in patients with osteoarthritic knee pain: a randomized controlled study. Pain 2004; 110: 539-49.

[28]   Hughes S, Seymour R, Campbell R, Pollak N, Huber G, Sharma L. Impact of the Fit and Strong Intervention on older adults with osteoarthritis. The Gerontologist 2004; 44(2): 217-28.

[29]   Thorstensson C, Roos E, Petersson I, Ekdahl C. Six-week high-intensity exercise program for middle-aged patients with knee osteoarthritis: a randomized controlled trial. BMC Musculosk Dis 2005; 6: 27.

[30]   Bennell K, Hinman R, Metcalf B, Buchbinder R, McConnell J, McColl G *et al.* Efficacy of physiotherapy management of knee joint osteoarthritis: a randomised double-blind placebo-controlled trial. Annals Rheum Dis 2005; 64: 906-12.

[31]   Huang M, Yang R, Lee C, Chen T, Wang M. Preliminary results of integrated therapy for patients with knee osteoarthritis. Arthritis Rheum 2005; 53: 812-20.

[32]   Hay E, Foster N, Thomas E, Peat G, Phelan M, yates H *et al.* Effectiveness of community physiotherapy and enhanced pharmacy review for knee pain in people aged over 55 presenting to primary care: pragmatic randomised trial. BMJ 2006; 333: 995-1004.

[33]   Mikesky A, Mazzuca S, Brandt K, Perkins S, Damush T, Lane K. Effects of strength training on the incidence and progression of knee osteoarthritis. Arthritis Rheum 2006; 55: 690-9.

[34]   Song R, Lee EO, Lam P, Bae SC. Effects of a Sun-style Tai Chi exercise on arthritic symptoms, motivation and the performance of health behaviors in women with osteoarthritis. Taehan Kanho Hakhoe Chi 2007; 37(2): 249-56.

[35]   Brismee JM, Paige RL, Chyu MC, Boatright JD, Hagar JM, McCaleb JA *et al.* Group and home-based tai chi in elderly subjects with knee osteoarthritis: a randomized controlled trial. Clin Rehabil 2007; 21(2): 99-111.

[36]   Doi T, Akai M, Fujino K, Iwaya T, Kurosawa H, Hayashi H *et al.* Effect of home exercise of quadriceps on knee osteoarthritis compared with nonsteroidal antiinflammatory drugs. Am J Phys Med Rehab 2008; 87: 258-69.

[37]   Aglamis B, Toraman N, Yaman H. The effect of a 12-week supervised multicomponent exercise program on knee OA in Turkish women. J Back Musculosk Rehab 2008; 21: 121-8.

[38]   Jan M, Lin C, Lin Y, Lin J, Lin D. Effects of weight-bearing versus nonweight-bearing exercise on function, walking speed, and position sense in participants with knee osteoarthritis: a randomized controlled trial. Arch Phys Med Rehab 2009; 90: 897-904.

[39]   Wang C, Schmid CH, Hibberd PL, Kalish R, Roubenoff R, Rones R *et al.* Tai Chi is effective in treating knee osteoarthritis: a randomized controlled trial. Arthritis Rheum 2009; 61(11): 1545-53.

[40]   Jenkinson CM, Doherty M, Avery AJ, Read A, Taylor MA, Sach TH *et al.* Effects of dietary intervention and quadriceps strengthening exercises on pain and function in overweight people with knee pain: randomised controlled trial. BMJ 2009; 339: b3170.

[41]   Bennell K, Hunt M, Wrigley T, Hunter D, McManus F, Hodges P *et al.* Hip strengthening reduces symptoms but not knee load in people with medial knee osteoarthritis and varus malalignment: a randomised controlled trial. Osteoarthritis Cart 2010; 18: 621-8.

[42]   Ettinger WH, Jr., Burns R, Messier SP, Applegate W, Rejeski WJ, Morgan T *et al.* A randomized trial comparing aerobic exercise and resistance exercise with a health education program in older adults with knee osteoarthritis. The Fitness Arthritis and Seniors Trial (FAST). JAMA 1997; 277(1): 25-31.

[43]   Evcik D, Sonel B. Effectiveness of a home-based exercise therapy and walking program on osteoarthritis of the knee. Rheumatol Int 2002; 22(3): 103-6.

[44]   Messier SP, Thompson CD, Ettinger WH. Effects of long-term aerobic or weight training regimens on gait in an older, osteoarthritic population. J Appl Biomech 1997; 13: 205-25.

[45]   Rejeski WJ, Lawrence RB, Ettinger W, Morgan T, Thompson C. Compliance to exercise therapy in older participants with knee osteoarthritis: implication for treating disability. Med Sci Sports Exerc 1997; 29(8): 977-85.

[46]   Minor MA, Hewett JE, Webel RR, Anderson SK, Kay DR. Efficacy of physical conditioning exercise in patients with rheumatoid arthritis and osteoarthritis. Arthritis Rheum 1989; 32(11): 1396-405.

[47]   Kovar PA, Allegrante JP, MacKenzie CR, Peterson MG, Gutin B, Charlson ME. Supervised fitness walking in patients with osteoarthritis of the knee. A randomized, controlled trial. Ann Intern Med 1992; 116: 529-34.

[48]   Peterson MGE, Kovar-Toledano PA, Otis JG, Allegrante JP, MacKenzie CR, Gutin B *et al.* Effect of a walking program on gait characteristics in patients with osteoarthritis. Arthritis Care Res 1993; 6(1): 11-6.

[49]   Anderson JJ, Felson DT. Factors associated with osteoarthritis of the knee in the first national Health and Nutrition Examination Survey (HANES I). Evidence for an association with overweight, race, and physical demands of work. Am J Epidemiol 1988; 128(1): 179-89.

[50]   Cicuttini FM, Baker JR, Spector TD. The association of obesity with osteoarthritis of the hand and knee in women: a twin study. J Rheumatol 1996; 23(7): 1221-6.

[51]   Cooper C, Snow S, McAlindon TE, Kellingray S, Stuart B, Coggon D *et al.* Risk factors for the incidence and progression of radiographic knee osteoarthritis. Arthritis Rheum 2000; 43(5): 995-1000.

[52]   Spector TD, Hart DJ, Doyle DV. Incidence and progression of osteoarthritis in women with unilateral knee disease in the general population: the effect of obesity. Ann Rheum Dis 1994; 53(9): 565-8.

[53]   Jordan K, Arden N, Doherty M, Bannwarth B, Bijlsma J, Dieppe P et al. EULAR recommendations 2003: an evidence based approach to the management of knee osteoarthritis: report of a task force of the Standing Committee for International Clinical Studies Including Therapeutic Trials (ESCISIT). Annals Rheum Dis 2003; 62: 1145-55.

[54]   Fitzgerald G, Oatis C. Role of physical therapy in management of knee osteoarthritis. Curr Opinion Rheumatol 2004; 16: 143-7.

[55]   Hortobagyi T, Garry J, Holbert D, Devita P. Aberrations in the control of quadriceps muscle force in patients with knee osteoarthritis. Arthritis Care Res 2004; 51: 562-9.

[56]   Childs J, Sparto P, Fitzgerald G, Bizzini M, Irrgang J. Alterations in lower extremity movement and muscle activation patterns in individuals with knee osteoarthritis. Clinical Biomech 2004; 19: 44-9.

[57]   Lewek M, Rudolph K, Snyder-Mackler L. Control of frontal plane laxity during gait in patients with medial compartment knee osteoarthritis. Osteoarthritis Cart 2004;12:745-51.

[58]   Felson DT, Gross KD, Nevitt MC, Yang M, Lane NE, Torner JC *et al.* The effects of impaired joint position sense on the development and progression of pain and structural damage in knee osteoarthritis. Arthritis Rheum 2009; 61(8): 1070-6.

[59]   Hurley M. Muscle dysfunction and effective rehabilitation of knee osteoarthritis: what we know and what we need to find out. Arthritis Care Res 2003; 49: 444-52.

[60]   Fitzgerald G, Childs J, Ridge T, Irrgang J. Agility and perturbation training for a physically active individual with knee osteoarthritis. Phys Ther 2002; 82: 372-82.

[61]   Hurley MV, Scott DL. Improvements in quadriceps sensorimotor function and disability of patients with knee osteoarthritis following a clinically practicable exercise regime. Brit J Rheumat 1998; 37: 1181-7.

[62]   Diracoglu D, Aydin R, Baskent A, Celik A. Effects of kinesthesia and balance exercises in knee osteoarthritis. J Clin Rheum 2005; 11(6): 303-10.

[63]   Lin D, Lin Y, Chai H, Han Y, Jan M. Comparison of proprioceptive functions between computerized proprioception facilitation exercise and closed kinetic chain exercise in patients with knee osteoarthritis. Clin Rheumatol 2007; 26(4): 520-8.

[64]   Lynn SK, Costigan PA. Changes in the medial-lateral hamstring activation ratio with foot rotation during lower limb exercise. J Elect Kin 2008 March epub.

[65]   Lee MS, Pittler MH, Ernst E. Tai chi for osteoarthritis: a systematic review. Clin Rheumatol 2008; 27(2): 211-8.

[66]   Callaghan MJ, Oldham J, Hunt J. An evaluation of exercise regimes for patients with osteoarthritis of the knee: a single-blind randomized controlled trial. Clinical Rehab 1995; 9(3): 213-8.

[67]   van Baar ME, Assendelft WJ, Dekker J, Oostendorp RA, Bijlsma JW. Effectiveness of exercise therapy in patients with osteoarthritis of the hip or knee: a systematic review of randomized clinical trials. Arthritis Rheum 1999; 42(7): 1361-9.

[68]   Rogind H, Bibow-Nielsen B, Jensen B, Moller HC, Frimodt-Moller H, Bliddal H. The effects of a physical training program on patients with osteoarthritis of the knees. Arch Phys Med Rehab 1998; 79: 1421-7.

[69]   Suomi R, Collier D. Effects of arthritis exercise programs on functional fitness and perceived activities of daily living measures in older adults with arthritis. Arch Phys Med Rehab2003; 84: 1589-94.

[70]   Hurley MV, Walsh NE. Effectiveness and clinical applicability of integrated rehabilitation programs for knee osteoarthritis. Curr Opin Rheumatol 2009; 21(2): 171-6.

[71]   Walsh NE, Mitchell HL, Reeves BC, Hurley MV. Integrated exercise and self-management programmes in osteoarthritis of the hip and knee: a systematic review of effectiveness. Phys Therapy Rev 2006; 11(4): 289-97.

[72]   Hurley MV, Walsh NE, Mitchell HL, Pimm TJ, Patel A, Williamson E *et al.* Clinical effectiveness of a rehabilitation program integrating exercise, self-management, and active coping strategies for chronic knee pain: a cluster randomized trial. Arthritis Rheum 2007; 57(7): 1211-9.

[73]   Hurley MV, Walsh NE, Mitchell HL, Pimm TJ, Williamson E, Jones RH *et al.* Economic evaluation of a rehabilitation program integrating exercise, self-management, and active coping strategies for chronic knee pain. Arthritis Rheum 2007; 57(7): 1220-9.

[74]   Jessep SA, Walsh NE, Ratcliffe J, Hurley MV. Long-term clinical benefits and costs of an integrated rehabilitation programme compared with outpatient physiotherapy for chronic knee pain. Physiotherapy 2009; 95(2): 94-102.

[75]   Schipplein OD, Andriacchi TP. Interaction between active and passive knee stabilizers during level walking. J Orthopaed Res 1991; 9: 113-9.

[76]   Zhao D, Banks S, Mitchell K, D'Lima D, Colwell C, Fregley B. Correlation between the knee adduction torque and medial contact force for a variety of gait patterns. J Orthopaed Res 2007; 25: 789-97.

[77]   Miyazaki T, Wada M, Kawahara H, Sato M, Baba H, Shimada S. Dynamic load at baseline can predict radiographic disease progression in medial compartment knee osteoarthritis. Ann Rheum Dis 2002; 61(7): 617-22.

[78]   Thorstensson C, Henriksson M, von Porat A, Sjodahl C, Roos E. The effect of eight weeks of exercise on knee adduction moment in early knee osteoarthritis - a pilot study. Osteoarthritis Cart 2007; 15: 1163-70.

[79]   Bennell KL, Hunt MA, Wrigley TV, Hunter DJ, McManus FJ, Hodges PW *et al.* Hip strengthening reduces symptoms but not knee load in people with medial knee osteoarthritis and varus malalignment: a randomised controlled trial. Osteoarthritis Cart 2010; 18(5): 621-8.

[80]   Foroughi N, Smith RM, Lange AK, Baker MK, Fiatarone Singh MA, Vanwanseele B. Lower limb muscle strengthening does not change frontal plane moments in women with knee osteoarthritis: A randomized controlled trial. Clin Biomech (Bristol, Avon) 2010.

[81]   Brandt KD, Heilman DK, Slemenda C, Katz BP, Mazzuca SA, Braunstein EM *et al.* Quadriceps strength in women with radiographically progressive osteoarthritis of the knee and those with stable radiographic changes. J Rheumatol 1999; 26: 2431-7.

[82]   Tak E, Staats P, Van Hespen A, Hopman-Rock M. The effects of an exercise program for older adults with osteoarthritis of the hip. J Rheumatol 2005; 32(6): 1106-13.

[83]   Fransen M, Nairn L, Winstanley J, Lam P, Edmonds J. Physical activity for osteoarthritis management: a randomized controlled clinical trial evaluating hydrotherapy or Tai Chi classes. Arthritis Rheum 2007; 57(3): 407-14.

[84]   Hopman-Rock M, Westhoff MH. The effects of a health educational and exercise program for older adults with osteoarthritis for the hip or knee. J Rheumatol 2000; 27(8): 1947-54.

[85]   Ravaud P, Giraudeau B, Logeart I, Larguier J, Rolland D, Treves R *et al.* Management of osteoarthritis (OA) with an unsupervised home based exercise programme and/or patient administered tools. A cluster randomised controlled trial with a 2x2 factorial design. Ann Rheum Dis 2004; 63: 703-8.

[86]   Fransen M, McConnell S, Hernandez-Molina G, Reichenbach S. Exercise for osteoarthritis of the hip. Cochrane Database Syst Rev 2009(3):CD007912.

[87] McNair PJ, Simmonds MA, Boocock MG, Larmer PJ. Exercise therapy for the management of osteoarthritis of the hip joint: a systematic review. Arthritis Res Ther 2009; 11(3):R98.

[88] Hernandez-Molina G, Reichenbach S, Zhang B, Lavalley M, Felson DT. Effect of therapeutic exercise for hip osteoarthritis pain: results of a meta-analysis. Arthritis Rheum 2008; 59(9): 1221-8.

[89] Zhang W, Doherty M, Leeb BF, Alekseeva L, Arden NK, Bijlsma JW et al. EULAR evidence based recommendations for the management of hand osteoarthritis: Report of a Task Force of the EULAR Standing Committee for International Clinical Studies Including Therapeutics (ESCISIT). Ann Rheum Dis 2007; 66(3): 377-88.

[90] van Baar ME, Dekker J, Oostendorp RA, Bijl D, Voorn TB, Lemmens JA *et al.* The effectiveness of exercise therapy in patients with osteoarthritis of the hip or knee: a randomized clinical trial. J Rheumatol 1998; 25(12): 2432-9.

[91] Foley A, Halbert J, Hewitt T, Crotty M. Does hydrotherapy improve strength and physical function in patients with osteoarthritis--a randomised controlled trial comparing a gym based and a hydrotherapy based strengthening programme. Ann Rheum Dis 2003; 62(12):1162-7.

[92] Rogers MW, Wilder FV. Exercise and hand osteoarthritis symptomatology: a controlled crossover trial. J Hand Ther 2009; 22(1): 10-7; discussion 9-20; quiz 18.

[93] Stamm TA, Machold KP, Smolen JS, Fischer S, Redlich K, Graninger W *et al.* Joint protection and home hand exercises improve hand function in patients with hand osteoarthritis: a randomized controlled trial. Arthritis Rheum 2002; 47(1): 44-9.

[94] Lefler C, Armstrong JW. Exercise in the treatment of osteoarthritis in the hands of the elderly. Clinical Kinesiology 2004; 58(2): 1-6.

[95] McCarthy C, Mills P, Pullen R, Roberts C, Silman A, Oldham J. Supplementing a home exercise programme with a class-based exercise programme is more effective than home exercise alone in the treatment of knee osteoarthritis. Rheumatology 2004; 43(7): 880-6.

[96] Jan MH, Lin JJ, Liau JJ, Lin YF, Lin DH. Investigation of clinical effects of high- and low-resistance training for patients with knee osteoarthritis: A randomized controlled trial. Phys Therapy 2008; 88(4): 427-36.

[97] Nelson ME, Rejeski WJ, Blair SN, Duncan PW, Judge JO, King AC *et al.* Physical activity and public health in older adults: recommendation from the American College of Sports Medicine and the American Heart Association. Med Sci Sports Exerc 2007; 39(8):1435-45.

[98] Farr JN, Going SB, Lohman TG, Rankin L, Kasle S, Cornett M *et al.* Physical activity levels in patients with early knee osteoarthritis measured by accelerometry. Arthritis Rheum 2008; 59(9): 1229-36.

[99] DeHaan MN, Guzman J, Bayley MT, Bell MJ. Knee osteoarthritis clinical practice guidelines -- how are we doing? J Rheumatol 2007; 34(10): 2099-105.

[100] Li L, Maetzel A, Pencharz J, Maguire L, Bombardier C, Team TCHaAPC. Use of mainstream nonpharmacologic treatment by patients with arthritis. Arthritis Care Res 2004; 51(2): 203-9.

[101] Holden MA, Nicholls EE, Hay EM, Foster NE. Physical therapists' use of therapeutic exercise for patients with clinical knee osteoarthritis in the United kingdom: in line with current recommendations? Phys Ther 2008; 88(10): 1109-21.

[102] Holden MA, Nicholls EE, Young J, Hay EM, Foster NE. UK-based physical therapists' attitudes and beliefs regarding exercise and knee osteoarthritis: findings from a mixed-methods study. Arthritis Rheum 2009; 61(11): 1511-21.

[103] Mazieres B, Thevenon A, Coudeyre E, Chevalier X, Revel M, Rannou F. Adherence to, and results of, physical therapy programs in patients with hip or knee osteoarthritis. Development of French clinical practice guidelines. Joint Bone Spine 2008; 75(5): 589-96.

[104] Marks R, Allegrante J. Chronic osteoarthritis and adherence to exercise: a review of the literature. J Aging Phys Activ 2005; 13: 434-60.

[105] McCarthy C, Mills P, Pullen R, Richardson G, Hawkins N, Roberts C *et al.* Supplementation of a home-based exercise programme with a class-based programme for people with osteoarthritis of the knees: a randomised controlled trial and health economic analysis. Health Technol Assess 2004;46:1-61.

[106] Campbell R, Evans M, Tucker M, Quilty B, Dieppe P, Donovan J. Why don't patients do their exercises? Understanding non-compliance with physiotherapy in patients with osteoarthritis of the knee. J Epidemiology Community Health 2001; 55: 132-8.

[107] Castro C, King A, Brassington G. Telephone versus mail interventions for maintenance of physical activity in older adults. Health Psychol 2001; 20: 438-44.

[108] Duncan K, Pozehl B. Effects of an exercise adherence intervention on outcomes in patients with heart failure. Rehab Nursing 2003; 28: 117-22.

[109] Litt M, Kleppinger A, Judge J. Initiation and maintenance of exercise behaviour in older women: predictors from the social learning model. J Behav Med 2002; 25: 83-97.

[110] Noland M. The effects of self-monitoring and reinforcement on exercise adherence. Res Q Exerc Sport 1989; 60: 212-24.

[111] Roddy E, Doherty M. Changing life-styles and osteoarthritis: what is the evidence? Best Practice & Research Clinical Rheumatology 2006; 20: 81-97.

[112] MacDonald CW, Whitman JM, Cleland JA, Smith M, Hoeksma HL. Clinical outcomes following manual physical therapy and exercise for hip osteoarthritis: A case series. J Orthop Sports Phys Ther 2006; 36(8): 588-99.

[113] French HP. Physiotherapy management of osteoarthritis of the hip: a survey of current practice in acute hospitals and private practice in the Republic of Ireland. Physiotherapy 2007; 93(4): 253-60.

[114] Walsh NE, Hurley MV. Evidence based guidelines and current practice for physiotherapy management of knee osteoarthritis. Musculoskeletal Care 2009; 7(1): 45-56.

[115] Moss P, Sluka K, Wright A. The initial effects of knee joint mobilization on osteoarthritic hyperalgesia. Man Ther 2007; 12(2): 109-18.

[116] Hoeksma HL, Dekker J, Ronday HK, Heering A, van der Lubbe N, Vel C et al. Comparison of manual therapy and exercise therapy in osteoarthritis of the hip: A randomized clinical trial. Arthritis Care Res 2004; 51(5): 722-9.

[117] Hoeksma HL, Dekker J, Ronday HK, Breedveld FC, Van den Ende CH. Manual therapy in osteoarthritis of the hip: outcome in subgroups of patients. Rheumatology (Oxford) 2005; 44(4): 461-4.

[118] Pollard H, Ward G, Hoskins W, Hardy K. The effect of a manual therapy knee protocol on osteoarthritic knee pain: a randomised controlled trial. JCCA J Can Chiropr Assoc 2008; 52(4): 229-42.

[119] Abbott JH, Robertson MC, McKenzie JE, Baxter GD, Theis JC, Campbell AJ. Exercise therapy, manual therapy, or both, for osteoarthritis of the hip or knee: a factorial randomised controlled trial protocol. Trials 2009; 10: 11.

[120] French HP, Cusack T, Brennan A, White B, Gilsenan C, Fitzpatrick M et al. Exercise and manual physiotherapy arthritis research trial (EMPART): a multicentre randomised controlled trial. BMC Musculoskelet Disord 2009; 10: 9.

[121] Deyle GD, Allison SC, Matekel RL, Ryder MG, Stang JM, Gohdes DD *et al.* Physical therapy treatment effectiveness for osteoarthritis of the knee: a randomized comparison of supervised clinical exercise and manual therapy procedures versus a home exercise program. Phys Ther 2005; 85(12): 1301-17.

[122] Deyle GD, Henderson NE, Matekel RL, Ryder MG, Garber MB, Allison SC. Effectiveness of manual physical therapy and exercise in osteoarthritis of the knee. A randomized, controlled trial. Ann Intern Med 2000; 132(3): 173-81.

[123] Perlman AI, Sabina A, Williams AL, Njike VY, Katz DL. Massage therapy for osteoarthritis of the knee: a randomized controlled trial. Arch Intern Med 2006; 166(22): 2533-8.

[124] Field T, Diego M, Hernandez-Reif M, Shea J. Hand arthritis pain is reduced by massage therapy. J Bodywork Mov Ther 2007; 11(1): 21-4.

CHAPTER 6

Components of Crenobalneotherapy for Knee Osteoarthritis: A Systematic Review

R. Forestier* and A. Françon

Centre de recherche rhumatologique et thermale, 15, avenue Charles de Gaulle, 73100 Aix-les-Bains, France.

Abstract: This chapter reports on a systematic review of the literature of crenobalneotherapy in the management of knee OA. Crenobalneotherapy is defined as the spectrum of techniques based on mineral or tap water and its derivatives, as used in a medical context. We searched Medline using the following keywords: "spa therapy", "mud", "radon", "balneotherapy", and "hydrotherapy" in combination with "OA", "arthrosis", and "gonarthrosis". We also reviewed the reference lists of articles retrieved by the Medline search. All studies that compared crenobalneotherapy to any other intervention or to no intervention were selected, and a checklist was used to assess their internal validity, external validity and the quality of the statistical analysis. We analyzed separately some components of crenobalneotherapy and comparators and four types of outcome criteria (pain, function, stiffness and quality of life). We calculated standardized response mean. There is middle level evidence that "multiple mineral interventions" that combine two or more components of crenobalneotherapy are superior to no treatment, high level evidence that its combination with home exercises is superior to home exercises alone and low level evidence that it is superior to short wave. There is high level but conflicting evidence that water exercise is superior to no treatment. There is a high level of evidence that water exercise is similar to land based exercise (but the studies noted that it is better tolerated). There is middle level evidence that massage is superior to no treatment. There is low level and conflicting evidence that bathing in mineral water is superior to or similar to bathing in tap water and that mineral mud and bathing in mineral water is superior to hot water. The only study evaluating heat (heat sleeve vs regular sleeve) found no differences but was a pilot study with insufficient sample size. Crenobalneotherapy seems to improve, pain, function, stiffness and quality of life in lower limb OA. As a whole treatment, its efficacy has a high level of evidence but efficacy of each component has middle level (massage) and sometimes high but conflicting level of evidence (exercise in water). There is low level evidence that chemical composition of water has a clinical relevant effect. More studies with higher methodology quality and sufficient sample size are needed in these fields.

Keywords: OA, validity, crenobalneotherapy, balneotherapy, hydrotherapy, massage, water exercise, mineral water, balneology.

1. INTRODUCTION

Limb osteoarthritis (OA) is an extremely common disease the prevalence of which increases with age. Although the exact prevalence of limb OA in France is unknown, a survey established that 14.8% of the rheumatologist visits were due to limb OA, compared to 13.7% due to OA of the spine [1].

Limb OA has a major impact on the everyday life of affected patients and imposes heavy costs on public healthcare services [2]. The direct cost of OA was estimated at 1.6 billion euros in France in 2002 [3], with half of this cost being ascribable to hospital care. OA required 13 million physician visits and 570 million euros worth of drugs. Management costs of OA increased by 156% compared to 1993 as a result of both a 54% increase in patient numbers and a 2.5% increase in annual cost per patient [3]. Although this study included OA at all sites, the high prevalence of limb OA indicates a substantial contribution to total costs. Literature reviews and clinical practice guidelines are available for knee OA. Among them, the most widely used are the recommendations issued by the Osteoarthritis Research Society International (OARSI) [4]. The

*Address correspondence to R. Forestier: Centre de recherche rhumatologique et thermal, 15, avenue Charles de Gaulle, 73100 Aix-les-Bains, France; Tel: +31 4 79 35 14 87; Fax: +31 4 79 34 16 15.; E-mail: romain.forestier@wanadoo.fr

Yves Henrotin, Kim Bennell and Francois Rannou (Eds)

expert panel did not gave a role for crenobalneotherapy but recommend some components that can be delivered in a spa centre, especially in recommendation 5: "For patients with symptomatic hip OA, exercises in water can be effective" and 10: "Some thermal modalities may be effective for relieving symptoms in hip and knee OA".

Crenobalneotherapy for limb OA is nevertheless widely used in France [5] and in other countries in Europe, North Africa, Middle East and Asia. We propose this term over narrower terms such as "balneotherapy" or "hydrotherapy", as the various therapeutic uses of water and its derivatives are sufficiently similar to be dealt with together. "Balneotherapy" includes use of tap water in south of Europe and mineral water in northern Europe. The root "creno" is derived from the Greek "crenos" that mean noun of mineral water. We define crenobalneotherapy as the spectrum of techniques based on mineral or tap water and its derivatives, as used in a medical context. Crenobalneotherapy includes many components, whose effects may be additive. These components include mud-packs, steam, water jets, and mobilization or hydromassages in a pool; physical effects related to heat pressure and massages; chemical effects of the water and its derivatives; and the effects of being away from home and following the spa lifestyle. They can be evaluated altogether as a complex strategy or separately but there are only a few similarities with evaluation of drugs because blinding is impossible for most of the components except chemical composition of the mineral water.

The objective of this study was to conduct a systematic literature review of studies that evaluated medical spa therapy in patients with OA of the knee and/or hip. We used the data to discuss the possible role for medical spa therapy in patients with these conditions.

2. METHODS

2.1. Search Strategy

We conducted a literature search in December 2009. Medline was searched using the terms "OA" AND "spa therapy" OR "mud" OR "balneotherapy"OR "hydrotherapy" OR "radon") AND ((clinical[Title/Abstract] AND trial[Title/Abstract]) OR clinical trials[MeSH Terms] OR clinical trial[Publication Type] OR random*[Title/Abstract] OR random allocation[MeSH Terms] OR therapeutic use[MeSH Subheading]). For each article retrieved using our search terms, we looked for additional articles by using the related article link on Medline, reviewing Medline articles by the same authors as the retrieved article, and reviewing the reference list of the retrieved article.

2.2. Selection of Articles

All studies that compared medical spa therapy to other interventions or to no intervention were considered. We also considered massage, heat and water exercises that are regularly used in spa centres. Only studies of patients with OA of the knee and/or hip written in English or French were studied.

2.3. Assessment of the Methodological Quality of Retrieved Articles

To assess internal validity, we used a checklist specifically designed for non-pharmacological trials (CLEAR NPT, [6]). Its items were selected using the Delphi method to develop a consensus among 55 experts. At present, there is no universally accepted checklist for evaluating the methodological quality of non-pharmacological trials in which the possible influence of multiple sources of bias raises specific challenges [7]. The external validity of each study was assessed to determine whether the source population was clearly defined and what proportion of screened patients with the disease was included in the analysis. To assess the quality of the statistical analysis, we used four criteria: whether parametric tests were used for normally distributed data and nonparametric tests otherwise, whether the study design provided adequate control of Type I error (risk of erroneously rejecting the null hypothesis) and Type II error (risk of erroneously accepting the null hypothesis), and whether between-group differences were clearly reported.

Arbitrarily, we defined total validity scores between 16 and 14 as high level evidence, between 13 and 11 as middle level evidence and less than 11 as low level evidence.

2.4. Magnitude of the Treatment Effect

As it is difficult to use a placebo intervention in crenobalneotherapy most of the trials compare crenobalneotherapy or its components with other active treatment, or sometimes with no treatment. We calculated separately standardized response means for different components of crenobalneotherapy (bath in mineral water, exercise in tap water, heat sleeve, massage, mineral mud or "multiple mineral intervention" when more than one component is evaluated in the trial) and different comparators (bath in tap water, depleted mud, drug therapy, home exercise, land based exercises, no treatment, regular sleeve or telephone call).

We chose between two methods for estimating the magnitude of the treatment effect, based on the data available in the article. In the first one, it was computed as the difference between the mean initial value and mean follow up over the standard deviation (SD) of the initial value. Alternatively, we computed the Standardized Response Mean (SRM) as the mean score change over the SD of that change [8]. The SRM was computed for pain, function, stiffness and quality-of-life indices, according to all available data. SRM values smaller than 0.3 are taken to indicate a negligible effect, values between 0.3 and 0.5 a small effect, values between 0.5 and 0.8 a moderate effect, and values greater than 0.8 a large effect. Correlations were evaluated using Spearman's r coefficient for nonparametric samples.

2.5. Estimation of Publication Bias

To estimate publication bias we used the empirical graphical method suggested by Sutton *et al.* [9] relating real distribution of SRM (on X axis) with sample size of crenobalneotherapy component and comparing it with a normal distribution (on Y axis). We combined SRM for pain, function, stiffness and quality of life that we consider as relevant outcome criteria for OA. As SRM can be quite different according to different follow up we calculated publication bias between 12 and 26 weeks which is a relevant follow up for a chronic disease.

3. RESULTS

Fig. **1** shows the results of the article selection procedure. We identified 236 assessable articles on which we analyzed 27 trials, including 17 undertaken in spa-therapy centers [10-26] with mineral water and 10 in non spa therapy centers [27-36].

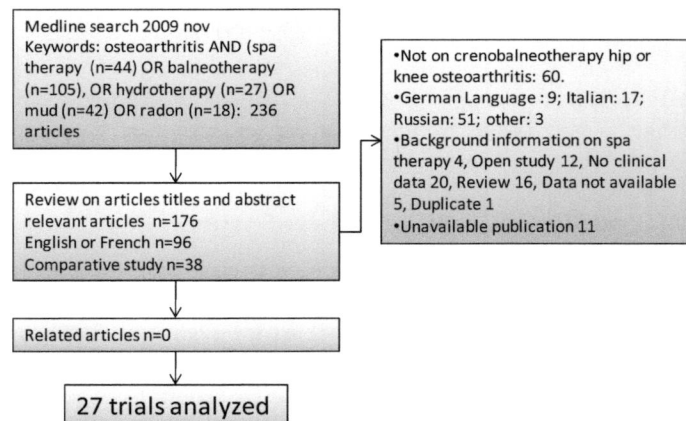

Figure 1: Flow chart of selection articles.

3.1. Evaluation of Study Methodologies

Table **1** reports the internal validity of the selected studies and Table **2** the results regarding the quality of statistical analyses and external validity. The statistical tests were usually appropriate for the distribution of the data. In some of the trials, Type I error control was inadequate, because no primary evaluation criterion

Table 1: Internal validity of the selected studies.

Method / Study: *Number of Positive item*	1 : adequate randomization	2 : concealed allocation	3 : description of the interventions	4 : experienced therapists	5 : compliance of the participants	6 : blinded patients or similar concomitants treatments, withdrawal and lost to follow up rates	7 : therapist blinded or similar concomitants treatments, withdrawal and lost to follow up rates	8 : Investigator blinded; or measures to avoid bias	9 : Same schedule in the two groups	10 : Intention to treat analysis
Balint 2006: *6/10*	Yes	No	Yes	Not reported, but probable (spa centre)	Not reported	Yes	No But similar concomitants treatments, withdrawal and lost to follow up rates	Yes	Yes	Not reported
Cantariti 2007: *3/10*	No	No	Yes	Not reported but probable (spa centre)	Not reported	No	Not reported	Not reported	Yes	Not reported
Cochrane 2005 a: *4/10*	Not randomized	No	Yes	Yes	Yes	No, similar concomitant treatment but more lost to follow up in st group	Not reported, similar concomitant treatment but more lost to follow up in st group	No : self-question-naire	Yes	No
Cochrane 2005 b: *8/10*	Yes	Yes	Yes	Yes	Yes	No	No	Yes	Yes	Yes
Evcik 2006: *3/10*	Not reported	Not reported	Yes	Not reported but probable (spa centre)	Not reported	No, concomitants treatment evaluated but not reported, lost to follow up Not reported.	Not reported, concomitants treatment evaluated but not reported, lost to follow up Not reported.	Not reported	Yes	Not reported
Fioravanti 2009: *7/10*	Yes	Not reported	Yes	Not reported but probable (spa centre)	Not reported	No but similar concomitants treatments, withdrawal and lost to follow up rates	No but similar concomitants treatments, withdrawal and lost to follow up rates	No : self-question-naire	Yes	Yes
Flusser 2002: *5/10*	Not reported	Not reported	Yes	No (self treatment)	No	Yes	Yes	Yes	Yes	No
Foley 2003: *9/10*	Yes	Yes	Yes	Yes	Yes	No	Yes	Yes	Yes	Yes
Forestier 2000: *4/10*	Not randomized	No	Yes	Yes	Yes	No ; similar concomitant treatment but different lost to follow up	Yes	No	No	No
Forestier 2009: *8/10*	Yes	Yes	Yes	Yes	No	Yes	Yes	no, independent investigator but self question-naire	Yes	Yes
Fransen 2007: *9/10*	Yes	Yes	Yes	Yes	Yes	Yes	Not reported	Yes	Yes	Yes
Green 1993: *5/10*	Not reported	Not reported	Yes	Not reported but probable	Yes	Non	Not reported	Yes	Yes	No
Hinman 2007: *8/10*	Yes	Yes	Yes	Yes	Yes	Not reported	Not reported	Yes	Yes	Yes
Karagulle 2007: *7/10*	Yes	Yes	Yes	Not reported but probable	Not reported	Not reported	Not reported	Yes	Yes	Yes

Kovacs 2002: 6/10	Yes	Yes	Yes	Not reported, but probable	Not reported	Yes	Not reported	Yes	Not reported	No
Lundt 2008: 7/10	Yes	Yes	Yes	Yes	Not reported	No, concomitant treatments not reported, difference in lost to follow up (20% in land based, 3% in aquatic)	Not reported, concomitant treatments not reported, difference in lost to follow up (20% in land based, 3% in aquatic)	Yes	Yes	Yes
Mazzuca 2004: 8/10	Yes	Not reported	Yes	Not relevant	Yes	Yes	Not relevant	Yes	Yes	Not reported
Nguyen 1997: 5/10	Yes	Not reported	Yes	Not reported, but probable	Not reported	No	Not reported	Yes	Yes	No
Obadasi 2002: 6/10 (knee)	Not randomized	No	Yes	Not reported but probable	Not reported	No but similar concomitant treatment	No but similar concomitant treatment	Yes	Yes	No
Patrick 2001: 5/10	Yes	Not reported	Yes	Yes	Yes	No. similar concomitants treatments, but different withdrawal and lost to follow up rates	No. similar concomitants treatments, but different withdrawal and lost to follow up rates	No : self question-naires	Yes	Not reported
Perlman 2006: 5/10	Yes	Not reported	Yes	Yes	Not reported	No	No	No : self question-naires	Yes	Yes
Sherman 2009: 7/10	Yes	Not reported	Yes	Not relevant	Not reported but probable	No. concomitants treatment not reported but similar lost to follow up	No. concomitants treatment not reported but similar lost to follow up	Yes	Yes	Yes (1 lost to follow up)
Silva 2008: 8/10	Yes	Not reported	Yes	Yes	Yes	No but similar concomitants treatments, withdrawal and lost to follow up rates	No but similar concomitants treatments, withdrawal and lost to follow up rates	No : self question-naires	Yes	Yes
Sukenik 1999 : 5/10	Not reported	Not reported	Yes	Not reported but probable	Not reported	Partial : blinding of the other treatment group	Not reported but similar concomitant treatment. lost to follow up Not reported	Yes	Yes	No
Szucs 1989: 4/10	Not reported	Not reported but independent	Yes	Not reported but probable	Not reported	Yes	Not reported	Not reported	Not reported	No
Tishler 2004: 5/10	Not reported	Yes	Yes	Not reported but probable	Yes	No	Not reported	No : self-question-naires	Yes	No
Vaht 2008: 3/10	Not randomized	No	Yes	Not reported but probable	Not reported	No	No	Not reported	Yes	Not reported
Wigler 1995: 5/10	Not reported	Not reported	Yes	Not reported but probable	Not reported	Yes	Not reported	Yes	Yes	No
Yurtkuran 2006 :4/10	Yes	Not reported	Yes	Not reported but probable	Not reported	No	Not reported	Yes	Not reported	No

was selected and/or because multiple criteria and measurements were used without adjusting the level of statistical significance. Type II error control was poor in some of the studies, so that results suggesting lack of efficacy may in fact have been due to lack of statistical power. Six randomized studies failed to report the results of between group comparisons, precluding confirmation of the study hypothesis. Half of the study reports described the proportion of evaluated patients who were included in the study. Fig. **2** shows that validity increased significantly between 1989 and 2009.

Table 2: Statistical and external validity of selected study.

Method Study: Number of Positive item	1 adapted statistical Tests	2 : control of Alpha risk	3 : control of Beta risk	4 : intergroup comparison	5 : defined or representative population	6 : number of analyzed patients/ randomized patients/number of screened patients
Balint 2006 : 2/6	Yes	Yes	No	No	Not reported	52/?/??
Cantariti 2007: 1/6	No: T test for group of 20 patients	No	No	Yes	No	74/ 74/?
Cochrane 2005 a: 6/6	Yes	Yes	Yes	Yes	Yes	60/125 40/ ?
Cochrane 2005 b: 6/6	Yes	Yes	Yes	Yes	Yes : population of osteoarthritis and press announcement	147/312
Evcik 2006: 2/6	Yes	No	No	Yes	Not reported	80/ ?
Fioravanti 2009: 4/6	Yes	No	No	Yes	Yes: outpatients in rheumatology unit	80/112
Flusser 2002: 3/6	Yes	No	No	yes	No	58/?/?
Foley 2003: 3/6	Yes	No	No	Yes	Not reported	105/429
Forestier 2000: 5/6	Yes	Yes	No	Yes	Yes : real population of patient	73/136
Forestier 2009:6/6	Yes	Yes	Yes	Yes	Yes press announcement, medical office, pharmacies…	382/630
Fransen 2007: 6/6	Yes	Yes	Yes	Yes	Yes press announcement, medical office, pharmacies, associations…	152/637
Green 1993: 4/6	Doubtful : analysis of variance on groups < 30	Yes	No	Yes	Yes : institution patients	43/67
Hinman 2007: 6/6	Yes	Yes	Yes	Yes	Yes: press announcement, medical office, pharmacies…	71/312
Karagulle 2008: 4/6	Yes	No: multiple measures and outcome	No	Yes	Yes: Outpatient Clinic for Rheumatic Diseases	20/100
Kovacs 2002: 2/6	Yes	No : multiples measures and judgment criteria	No	No	Not reported	58/70
Lund 2008: 6/6	Yes	Yes	Yes	Yes	Outpatient clinic, general practitioner, local newspaper	70/184

Mazzuca 2004: 4/6	Yes	No	No	Yes	Not reported	51/?
Nguyen 1997: 5/6	Yes	Yes	Yes	Yes	Not reported	93/117
Obadasi 2002: 4/6	Yes	Yes	Yes	Yes	Not reported	49/ ?
Patrick 2001: 5/6	Yes	Yes	Yes	Yes	Yes : press announcement	249/ ?
Perlman 2006: 5/6	Yes	No: 7 outcome for p<0.05 but with Bonferroni correction significant p<0.007 is achieved fo 3/7 criteria	Yes	Yes	Yes: Outpatient clinic	53/210
Sherman 2009: 1/6	No: t test on group of 20 patients	No: 6 outcome and 3 measures for p<0,05	No	No	Yes: Outpatient clinic	44/?
Silva 2008: 5/6	Yes	Yes	Yes	Yes	Yes: Outpatient clinic	57/?
Sukenik 1999: 1/6	Doubtful : t test on groups of 10 patients	Yes	No	No	Not reported	40/ ?
Szucs 1989: 2/6	Not reported	No : 5 criteria and 3 measures for p<0,05	No	Yes	Not reported	62/ ?
Tishler 2004: 4/6	Yes	No : 5 criteria and 3 measures for p<0,05	No	No	Yes : press announcement	72/136
Vaht 2007: 3/6	Yes	No	No	Yes	Yes: sample of patient arriving for spa treatment	296/?
Wigler 1995: 0/6	No : ANOVA and t test for groups of 10 patients	No : 7 criteria et 8 measures pour p<0,05	No	No	Not reported	33/ ?
Yurtkuran 2006: 5/6	Yes	Yes	No	Yes	Yes by telephone on osteoarthritis population well known of the centre	56/102

Alpha risk represents the risk to conclude erroneously to a difference between group. If it is not controlled, we cannot conclude to a statistical difference between interventions. Beta risk is the risk to conclude erroneously to equivalence between interventions. External validity determine in which measure the study is applicable in "real life". It depends of availability of treatment and representatives of studied patients.

Table **3** shows our conclusions based on our evaluation of the methodology and statistical analyses used in the selected studies.

3.2. Magnitude of the Treatment Effect

A meta-analysis was considered inappropriate given the considerable variations in the interventions used, control groups (most notably regarding the efficacy of the comparator intervention), evaluation criteria (pain, Lequesne index, WOMAC index and his components, quality-of-life indices), and follow-up duration (8 days to 18 months). The mean effect size has little relevance under these circumstances. We calculated the weighed magnitude of the treatment effect for the evaluated components in Table **4**. We attempted to estimate the relation between SRM and follow up for pain, function, stiffness and quality of life in Fig. **3** and the weighed SRM of the different components and comparators in Table **5**. There was no correlation between validity and SRM (r spearman: 0.09, p = 0.66).

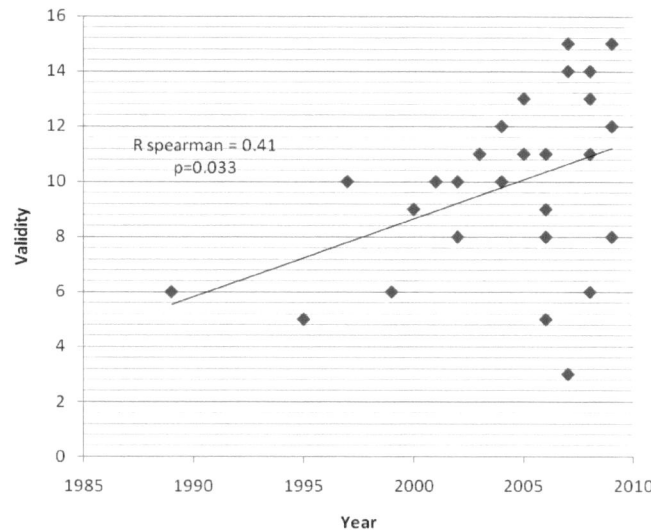

Figure 2: Correlation between year of publication and validity. Validity significantly improves with time.

3.3. Publication Bias

Estimation of publication bias is reported in Fig. **4** by a graphical test about relation between SRM and sample size. Fig. **3a** representing crenobalneotherapy components at all times indicate that publication bias probably overestimates SRM but it probably has a minimal influence on result if we keep only follow up between 12 and 26 weeks (Fig. **3b**).

3.4. Data Analysis and Interpretation

There is middle level evidence that "multiple mineral interventions" that combine 2 or more components of crenobalneotherapy are superior to no treatment [12, 18], high level evidence that combination with home exercises is superior to home exercises alone [15] and low level evidence that it is superior to short wave [11]. There is low level evidence (non randomized studies) that 16 sessions are superior to 2 sessions [19] and that 6 days of treatment is similar to 12 days [24].

There is high level but conflicting evidence that water exercise is superior to no treatment. Some trials find superiority [27, 28, 30, 32, 33], some others, usually with smaller sample size and smaller validity score, found no difference [29, 31, 34]. Hinman *et al.* suggest that type of exercise intervention (gradual, individually tailored, close supervision) can lead to a better result [31]. Others have found that the treatment effect was proportional to compliance, which declined gradually over time [27, 28]. There is a high level of evidence that water exercise is similar [31, 34] to land-based exercise (but the studies noted that water exercise is better tolerated). Most of the protocols used in these studies differed markedly from those used at medical spas that are usually limited from 1 to 4 weeks in duration.

There is middle level evidence that massage is superior to no treatment [35]. There is low level and conflicting evidence that bathing in mineral water is superior to [9, 17, 20-22, 25] or similar [26] to bathing in tap water and that mineral mud and bathing in mineral water is superior to hot packs [11]. Only two of these studies reported between group comparisons [20, 24].

The only study evaluating heat (heat sleeve vs regular sleeve) found no differences but was a pilot study with insufficient sample size [45].

When we examined the clinical effect of all crenobalneotherapy components, we estimate that there is an important effect for pain in the five first weeks, moderate effect between 5-50 weeks and a small effect after 50 weeks. For function, the effect is moderate between 0 and 30 weeks, small between 30 and 60 weeks and negligible later. The effect size for quality of life is moderate between 0 and 50 weeks and small later.

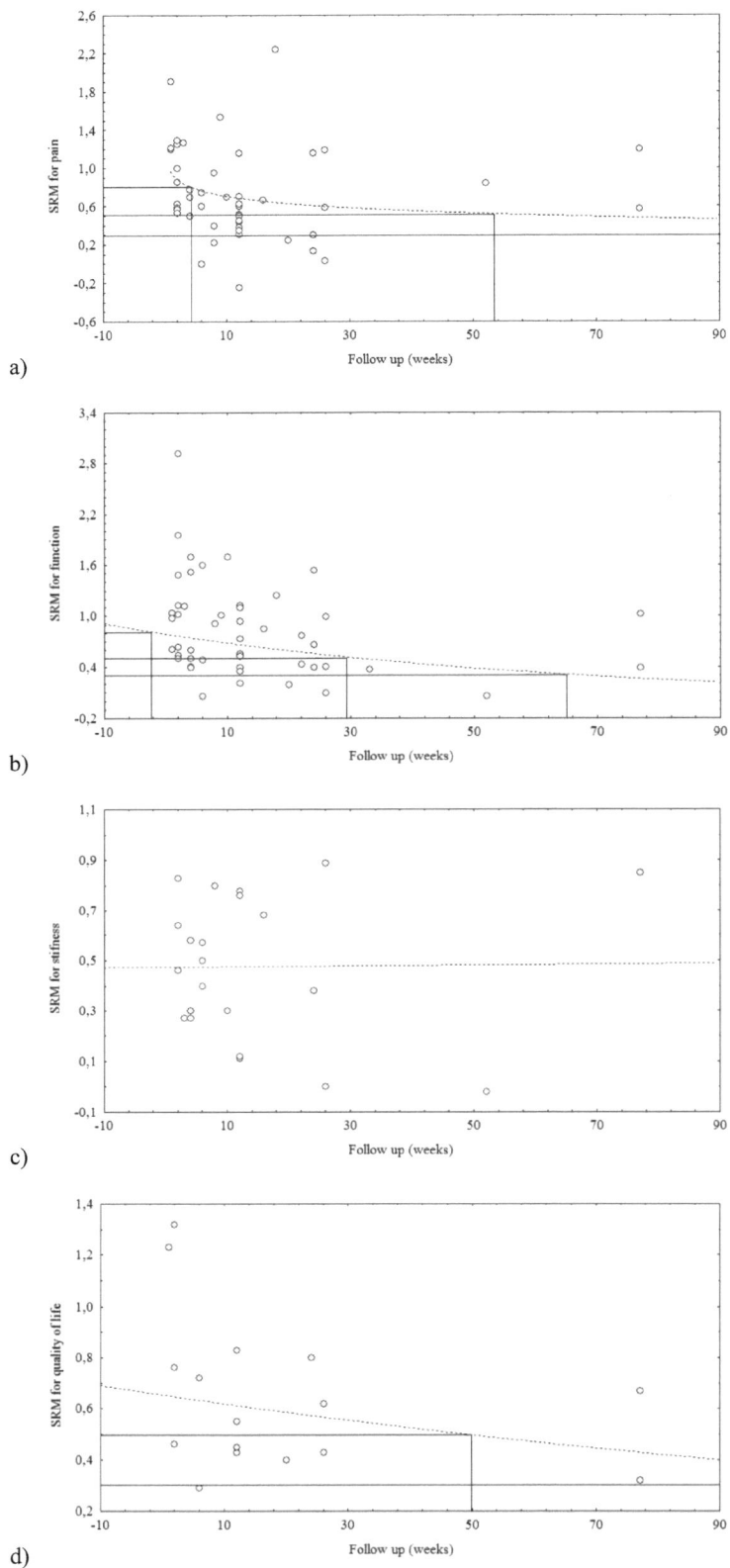

Figure 3: a) relation between SRM and follow-up for pain; b) relation between SRM and follow-up for function; c) relation between SRM and follow-up for stiffness; d) relation between SRM and follow-up for quality of life.

Table 3: Interpretation of trials.

Study	Our conclusions on selected study
Balint 2006	Statistical power was sufficient to detect an improvement versus baseline in the thermal mineral water group. Because the between-group difference was not computed, superiority of thermal mineral water over tap water cannot be confirmed.
Cantariti 2007	With major reservation for internal, external and statistical validity, the study is in favor of superiority of spa treatment on short wave and no treatment.
Cochrane 2005 a	Despite major reservations about internal validity, this pilot study showed that aquatic exercises were superior over no exercises.
Cochrane 2005 b	Internal validity, external validity, and statistical validity were good (the only missing feature was blinding of the patients and therapists). Improvements in quality-of-life and WOMAC indices were larger in the aquatic exercise group (1e2 sessions/week for 1 year) than in the usual-treatment group. The initial treatment effect was meaningful and comparable to other treatments, most notably drugs, used in osteoarthritis. Subsequently, the treatment effect was proportional to compliance, which declined gradually over time. Healthcare service utilization was reduced in the intervention group. The study was not powered to detect a cost/effectiveness difference between the two groups. Costs varied widely across patients, with joint replacement surgery and co-morbidity contributing large proportions of the total cost. Effects of the exercise program seemed similar in patients with knee and hip osteoarthritis.
Evcik 2006	Despite major reservations about internal validity, this study showed a longer pain-free walking distance with mud-pack therapy or balneotherapy than with hot-pack therapy. WOMAC index improvements were not different between the two groups.
Fioravanti 2009	With limited reservation about internal validity (lack of concealed allocation and compliance of participants, waiting list overestimate the difference between treatment and control group) statistical power is sufficient to detect that crenobalneotherapy is superior to no treatment (waiting list).
Foley 2003	Internal validity was good, but Type I and II error control was inadequate. Power was sufficient to establish that the WOMAC pain score and the quality-of-life SF12 physical summary score were higher in the hydrotherapy group than in the untreated controls. Power was inadequate to detect a difference between the hydrotherapy and gymnastic groups.
Forestier 2000	Despite reservations about internal validity, power was sufficient to detect significant and comparable improvements over both years. Because there was no control group, the placebo effect and the spa therapy effect cannot be separated. Two spa therapy treatments received at a 1-year interval by the same patients were compared, which probably introduced bias, as functional status was poorer during the second year.
Forestier 2009	With limited reservation on internal validity (compliance of participants) the study show that crenobalneotherapy plus home exercise is superior to exercise alone.
Fransen 2007	With limited reservation on internal validity (waiting list overestimate the difference between treatment and control group) this study shows that exercise in flat water is superior to no treatment.
Green 1993	Despite reservations about internal validity, power was sufficient to detect intragroup improvements versus baseline but not to detect a between-group difference.
Hinman 2007	Internal validity, external validity, and the statistical analysis were good. A clinically significant improvement was noted in the primary evaluation criterion (pain) in the aquatic physical therapy group (2e7 sessions/week for 20 weeks) compared to the group that continued usual treatment. The WOMAC index, muscle strength, and physical function also showed larger improvements. This study resembles the study by Patrick *et al.* [29] reported in 2001, and its authors ascribe the efficacy of their intervention to the more gradual and individually tailored nature of the exercises and to the close supervision of the patients (6 patients only per group).
Kovacs 2002	Power was sufficient to detect intragroup improvements versus baseline in both groups. The absence of between-group comparisons precludes conclusions about whether thermal water was superior over tap water.
Lund 2008	With some methodological limitation land based exercise seem to be superior and aquatic exercise similar to no treatment (low sample size, difference in lost to follow up exposing to an experimental mortality bias, lack of blinding of therapists, overestimation of difference with deception bias in the control group, some dropout in land based exercise group could be related to increase in pain that overestimate the treatment effect, mild difference in baseline value for pain can create a regression to mean bias for the main criteria change in pain).
Mazzuca 2004	With some methodological limitation (pilot study) the statistical power is sufficient to detect an improvement versus baseline but not sufficient to detect a superiority of the heat retaining knee sleeve.
Nguyen 1997	Despite reservations about internal validity, the study showed that spa therapy was better than continuing the usual treatment, regarding medication use (primary evaluation criterion), the Lequesne algofunctional index, and pain.
Obadasi 2002	Several methodological weaknesses were noted (absence of randomization leaving room for unrecognized sources of bias, compliance of the participants, intention-to-treat analysis). Combining mud packs and hydrotherapy was superior over two hydrotherapy sessions. The short time to evaluation, regression toward the mean and small sample size may have contributed to the unusually large treatment effect.

Patrick 2001	Despite a few reservations regarding the methodology (blinding of the patients, differences in dropout rates), the study established that hydrotherapy provided no clinical or medicoeconomic benefits compared to continuing the usual treatment. The exercise program used in this study seems to provide no medical or financial benefits.
Perlman 2006	Some methodological limitations: lack of concealed allocation, compliance of participants, blinding of patients and therapists, difference in lost to follow up (32% in the treatment group, 11% in the control group), évaluation of concomitants treatment may partly explain the differences between massage and waiting list. Waiting list may overestimate difference between treatment and control group.
Sherman 2009	High type I and type II error, some internal validity limitations and absence of between-group comparisons preclude conclusions from this study.
Silva 2008	Statistical power is sufficient do detect an intragroup improvement for all judgment criteria but insufficient to detect difference between hydrotherapy and land based exercises.
Sukenik 1999	The methodological weaknesses, low statistical power, absence of sample size estimation, and absence of between-group comparisons preclude conclusions from this study.
Szucs 1989	Despite reservations about the methodology and high risk of Type I error, the study had sufficient statistical power to show that thermal water was superior over tap water.
Tishler 2004	The difference in the number of patients in the treatment group (n ¼ 48) and control group (n ¼ 24) may be sufficient to explain the significant improvement in the treatment group but not in the controls. The absence of between-group comparisons precludes conclusions from this study.
Vaht 2007	With a lot of methodological limitations this study found no differences between a 6 an 12 days course of spa therapy.
Wigler 1995	The methodological weaknesses, high Type I error risk, and absence of between-group difference calculations preclude conclusions.
Yurkturan 2006	Reservations are in order regarding internal validity, and power was inadequate to detect a difference between thermal water and tap water regarding the primary evaluation criterion. Significant differences were noted for quadriceps strength and one of the five dimensions of the Nottingham Health Profile. Both groups showed improvements versus baseline for most of the evaluation criteria.

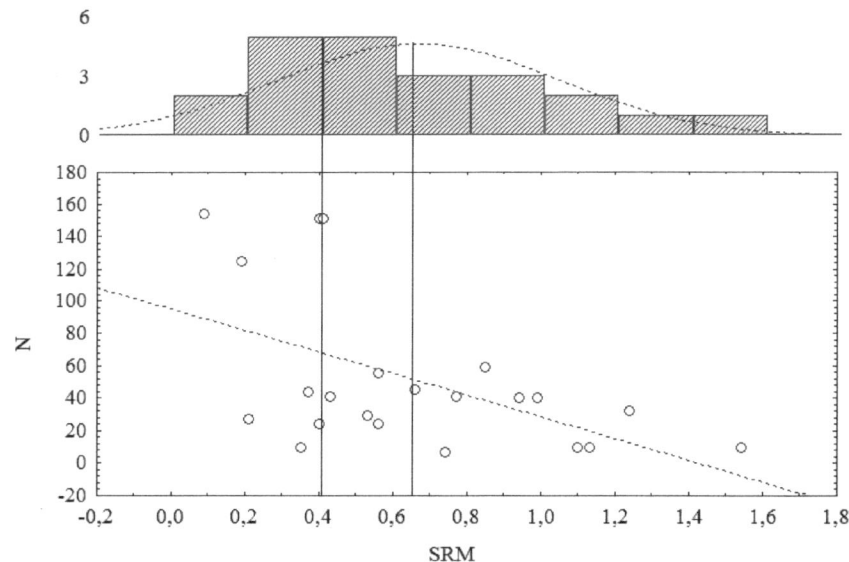

Figure 4: Relation between SRM and sample size between 12 & 26 weeks.

We are aware that a number of relevant studies were not included in our review. Some studies were published in journals that were not available for this review [36-47]. Furthermore, Medline does not include all published articles. Although high-quality studies are usually believed to appear in English-language peer-reviewed journals, valuable work may be reported in other languages.

An original feature of our study is that we used a checklist that was specifically designed to evaluate the internal validity of nonpharmacological trials. This checklist has been validated by a panel of experts. In addition, we assessed the statistical data handling and external validity of the studies, although no validated tools were available for these assessments. This is also the first study to evaluate publication bias and that estimates treatment effect along time and for different components of crenobalneotherapy.

A major obstacle to achieving a synthesis on crenobalneotherapy is the considerable variability of the interventions used. Thus, studies may compare spa products, spa care procedures, the global spa therapy strategy, chemical properties or aquatic exercises to a variety of other interventions. In addition, patients usually continue their usual medications during their stay at the spa. A few studies report a clinically relevant improvement for patients . We believe that future studies should include a qualitative criterion to determine whether improvements are perceived by the patients. In addition, a qualitative criterion would help to distinguish the placebo effect from the specific effect of medical spa therapy, as the placebo effect does not significantly influence discontinuous variables such as qualitative criteria [50].

Table 4: Standardized response mean.

Trial Year *Follow up*	Treatment	N	Judgment criteria	Improving with time	Between-group comparison	SRM
Balint 2006 *3 months*	Mineral water 34° : 30'/day during 20 days	27	WOMAC	1,29 +/-2,91	Not reported	*+0,44*
	Tap water 43° : 30'/day during 20 days	25		0 +/-3,32		*0*
Cochrane 2005 a *4 months*	Exercise in water 29° : 2 sessions of 1h/week during 3months	59	WOMAC pain	10,2 +/-3,25 → 7,54	S with control	+1,34
	Control (no exercise)	39		9,5 +/-3,75 → 9,3		+0,12
Cochrane 2005 b *1 year*	Exercise in water 29° : 2 sessions of 1h/week during 3 months	154	WOMAC pain	8,72 +/-3,62 → 8,46	S with control	+0,84
			WOMAC function	30,06 +/-13,13 → 29,26	NS	+0,06
			WOMAC limitation	3,86 +/-1,66 → 3,88	NS	-0,02
	Control (no exercise)	152	WOMAC pain	9,1 +/-3,14 → 9,35		-0,10
			WOMAC function	31,5 +/-11,24 → 32,42		-0,08
			WOMAC limitation	4,03 +/-1,42 → 4,15		0,02
Evcik 2006 *3 months*	Mineral water 36° : 10 sessions of 20'/day in 10 days	25	WOMAC	9,1 +/-3,6 → 7,5	NS	0,44
			Pain	719 +/-577 → 1064	S with hot pacs	0,60
	Mineral mud 42° : 10 sessions of 20'/day in 10 days	29	WOMAC	11 +/-3,3 → 9	NS	0,60
			Pain	442 +/-426 → 454	NS	0,02
	Hot packs 42° : 10 sessions of 20'/day in 10 days	26	WOMAC	9,9 +/-4,4 → 9,4		0,12
			Pain	668 +/-1085 → 740		0,08
Fioravanti 2009 9 months	Mud packs and bicarbonate sulfate mineral water	40	WOMAC pain	36.54 +/-13.8→ 20.53	S with control	1.19
			WOMAC function	37.65 +/-22.9→ 18.8		0.94
			AIMS	1.58 +/-1.07→ 0.99		0.55
	Control (waiting list)	40	WOMAC pain	36.82 +/- 15.77→ 38.13		-0.08
			WOMAC function	44.55 +/-18.86→ 43.45		0.06
			AIMS	1.69 +/-0.97→ 1.41		0.29

Forestier 2000 *5 months*	Spa therapy : massages, pool, mud, heat & shower : 18 sessions in 3 weeks	51	Lequesne	-1,7 +/-2,2	NS	*+0,76*
	spa therapy : massages, pool, mud, heat & shower : 18 sessions in 3 weeks	51		-1,3 +/-3		*+0.44*
Fransen 2007 12 weeks	Hydrotherapy : exercise in water, one hour, twice a week, 12 weeks	55	WOMAC pain	10,9 [6,5-15,3]	NS	
			Womac function	11,4 [6,3-16,6]	S with control	+0.63
	Control (waiting list)	41	WOMAC pain	4,4 [0,2-8,6]		
			Womac function	0,9 [-3,6-5,4]		
Hinman 2007 *6 months*	Exercise in water 34° : 12 sessions d'1h/day in 6 weeks	36	WOMAC	105,8 +/-45,2 → 81,4	NS	+0,74
			Pain	6 +/-2 → 4	S with control	+1,0
	Control (no Exercise)	35	WOMAC	92,9 +/-44,8 → 94,9		-0,04
			Pain	5 +/-2 → 5		0
Karagulle 2007	2 session mineral water 30' a day, holyday atmosphere in 10 days	10	Lequesne index			
			Pain			+0,60
	Usual care	10	Lequesne index			
			Pain			
Kovaks 2002 *3months*	Mineral water 36° : 30'/day in 15 days	31	Pain	-29 +/-120	Not reported	*+0,24*
	Eau courante 36° : 30'/j en 15j	27		-29 +/-77		*+0,36*
Lund 2008 3 months	Aquatic exercise 33.5°, two sessions of 20' a week, 8 weeks	26	Pain at rest	-11.7	NS	*+0.49*
			Pain during walking	-6.9	NS	*+0.37*
	Land-based exercise two sessions of 20' a week, 8 weeks	20	Pain at rest	-7.7	Significant with control	*+0.40*
			Pain during walking	-2.9	NS	*+0.14*
	Control (waiting list?)	24	Pain at rest	+8.3		*-0.41*
			Pain during walking	+9.8		*-0.30*
Mazzuca 2004 4 week	Heat retaining sleeve	26	Womac pain	-2.5 +/-3.2	NS	*+0.78*
			Womac stiffness	-0.5 +/-1.8		*+0.27*
			Womac function	-3.2 +/-7.8		*+0.41*
	Regular sleeve	25	Womac pain	-1.4 +/-1.8		*+0.77*
			Womac stiffness	-0.9 +/-1.5		*+0.60*
			Womac function	-4.2 +/-9.5		*+0.44*
Nguyen 1998 *6 months*	spa therapy : massages, pool, mud and shower: 18 sessions in 3 week	45	Pain	-9 +/-29	Significant with control	*+0,30*
			Lequesne	-2 +/-3		*+0,66*
			AIMS2	-0,4 +/-0,5	NS	*+0,80*
	usual care (waiting list)	48	Pain	+4 +/-26		*-0,14*
			Lequesne	0 +/-3		*0,00*
			AIMS2	+0,1 +/-1,1		*+0,10*
Obadasi 2002 8 days	bath in mineral water 39° : 20'/day + mineral mud 45° 20'/day in 8 days	24	Lequesne	-4,33 +/-2,17	S with 2nd treatment	*+1,98*
			Pain	-24,2 +/-10,4		*+2,32*
	2 bath 20'/j in Mineral water 39° in 8 days	25	Lequesne	-2,48 +/-1,18		*+2,10*
			Pain	-16,12 +/-6,37		*+2,52*
Patrick 2001	Exercise in water 42° : 2/s in 4 months	125	Quality of life	62,3 +/-16,9 → 65,8	S with control	*+0,20*
			HAQ	2,56 +/-1,13 → 2,31	NS	*+0,22*

		N				
5 months	no exercise	124	Quality of life	62,5 +/-16,7 → 61,7		*-0,04*
			HAQ	2,48 +/-1,12 → 2,58		*-0,09*
Perlman 2006 8 weeks	Massage 8 weeks	23	WOMAC pain	-23.19 +/-24.3	S with control	*+0.95*
			WOMAC function	20.50 +/- 22.5		*+0.91*
	waiting list 8 weeks)	30	WOMAC pain	-3.08 +/-17.5		*+0.17*
			WOMAC function	-0.02 +/-16.3		*0.00*
Sherman 2009 6 months	Sulphur pool 35°, 20' twice a week, 6 weeks	24	Pain	6.39 +/- 2.5 → 6.03	Not reported	*+0.14*
			WOMAC function	101.6 +/-33.6→88.3		*+0.13*
	Covered Jacuzzi 35°, 20' twice a week, 6 weeks	20	Pain	5.71 +/-2.47 →5.76		*-0.01*
			WOMAC function	99.6 +/-32.6 →86.1		*+0.13*
Silva 2008 18 weeks	Water-based exercises, 32° pool 50' session, 3/week, 18 week	31	Pain	61.9 +/-15.7→26.7	NS	*+2.24*
			WOMAC	32.8 +/-13.9 →15.6	NS	*+1.23*
	Land-based exercises, 50' session, 3/week, 18 week	26	Pain	68.2 +/-15.5 →37.3		*+1.99*
			WOMAC	34.9 +/-12.6 → 22.7		*+0.96*
Sukenik 1999 *3 months*	Sulphur pool 37° : 2/day in 12 days	10	Lequesne	15 +/-2,37 → 12	Not reported	+1,36
	bathing in the Dead sea: 2/day in 12 days	10		13 +/-2 → 12,1		+0,42
	Sulphur pool & bathing in the Dead Sea: 2/day in 12 days	10		13 +/-2.1 → 9,9		+1,40
	no balneotherapy 12 days	10		14,9 +/-1,9 → 14		+0,74
Tishler 2004 *10 weeks*	Mineral water : 37° : 1/week in 6 weeks	44	Pain	-38 +/-51	S with control	*+0,74*
			Lequesne	-4,8 +/-6		*+0,80*
			WOMAC	-16,8 +/-17		*+0,98*
	"usual care"	24	Pain	-4,2 +/-29		*+0,14*
			Lequesne	-1,2 +/-5		*+0,24*
			WOMAC	-3,8 +/- 26		*+0,14*
Vaht 2007 6&12 days	Mud treatment, pearl bath, shower massage, massage, therapeutic exercises 12 days	61	Pain	5.18 +/-1.7 → 2.9	NS	*+1.34*
			Lequesne	11.2 +/-3.7→ 7.2		*+1.08*
	Mud treatment, pearl bath, shower massage, massage, therapeutic exercises 6 days	235	Pain	5.59 +/-1.9 → 3.2		*+1.25*
			Lequesne	11.2 +/-3.7→ 7.5		*+1.00*
Yurtkuran 2006 *3 months*	Mineral water 37° : 20'/day 10 sessions in 2 weeks	27	WOMAC	60,35 +/-21,36 → 47	NS	*+0,62*
			Pain	53 +/-16,9 → 33		*+1,18*
	Tap water 37° : 20'/day 10 sessions in 2 weeks	25	WOMAC	65,9+/-13,6 → 47,3		*+1,36*
			Pain	61,1 +/-15,9 → 36		*+1,58*

N: analyzed patients, NS: not significant, S: significant. WOMAC: western Ontatio Mac Master University. AIMS: arthritis impact measurement scale. Ns: not significant. Improvement of patient corresponds with a decrease for some index (pain, Lequesne, WOMAC) and increase for some others (quality of life). For a better comprehension of the table, standardized response mean is noted positive when it is an improvement.

An obstacle to evaluations of medical spa therapy is that no satisfactory control group can be used. In most studies evaluating components, the effects are assessed compared to those on a waiting list.This is a better strategy than using untreated controls, which may have high dropout rates. However, it may lead to resentment among controls, with also increased dropout rates and deteriorating subjective clinical outcomes. One solution may be the randomization method suggested by Zelen [48, 49], in which patients are randomly divided into two groups, one of which receives standard treatment without being told that an experimental treatment is under study. Patients in the other group are asked whether they consent to experimental treatment; if they refuse, they are given standard treatment but are analyzed with the patients who accept, according to the intention-to-treat approach.

Table 5: Weighed standardized response mean of the different components (all judgment criteria) the components of crenobalneotherapy are reported in light grey and comparators in white.

Component\weeks	2	5	9	12	16	26	52	77
Multiple mineral intervention	1.19	0.60		0.50		0.52		0.46
Bath in mineral water	0.92	0.86	0.90	0.33		0.31		
Bath in sea	0.50	0.40		0.35				
Heat sleeve		0.49						
Massage			0.89					
Mineral mud	1.00			0.60				
Exercise in tap water		0.42	0.83	0.51	0.73	0.04	0.29	
Bath in tap water	0.49	0.33		0.35		0.08		
Home exercices				0.22		0.26		0.13
Land based exercise		0.03	0.83	0.36				
Depleted mud	0.47			0.12				
No treatment	-0.06	0.28	0.16	-0.04	0.05	-0.01	-0.05	0.22
Drug therapy	-0.34			-0.44		-0.21		
Regular sleeve		0.60						
Telephone call		-0.05						

CONCLUDING REMARKS

Crenobalneotherapy seems to improve, pain, function, stiffness and quality of life in lower limb OA. As a whole treatment, its efficacy has a high level of evidence but efficacy of each component has varying levels of evidence: *e.g.* middle level evidence for massage and sometimes high but conflicting levels of evidence for exercise in water. There is low evidence that chemical composition of water has a clinical relevant effect. More studies with higher methodology quality and sufficient sample size are needed.

ACKNOWLEDGEMENT

Some part of this chapter has been published previously in author's own manuscript entitled "Forestier R, Françon A. Crenobalneotherapyfor limb osteoarthritis: systematicliterature review and methodological analysis. Joint bone spine 2008; 75(2):138-48".

REFERENCES

[1]   La morbidité rhumatismale observée dans leur activité de consultation par les médecins rhumatologues appartenant au Réseau Epidémiologique de la Société Française de Rhumatologie (RESFR) Rev Rhum 1986; 53(5): 325-9.

[2]   Levy F, Ferme A, Perocheau D, Bono I. .Les coûts socio-économiques de l'arthrose en France. Rev Rhum 1993 ; 60: 63S-7S.

[3]   Le Pen C, Reygrobelet C, Gérentes I. Les conséquences socio-économiques de l'arthrose en France. Etude COART France. Rev Rhum 2005; 72: 1326-30.

[4]   Zhang W, Moskowitz RW, Nuki G, *et al.* OARSI recommendations for the management of hip and knee osteoarthritis, Part II: OARSI evidence-based, expert consensus guidelines. Osteoarthritis Cartilage 2008; 16: 137-62.

[5] Boulangé M., Guénot C., Fournier B., Gueguen R. Prévalence de la maladie rhumatismale et incidence du suivi des cures thermales chez les consultants âgés de 55 à 64 ans des Centres français d'examens de santé. Press Therm Clim 1999 ; 3: 149-56.

[6] Boutron I, Moher D, Tugwell P, *et al*. A checklist to evaluate a report of a nonpharmacological (CLEAR NTP) trial was developed using consensus. J Clin Epidemiol 2005; 58:1233-40.

[7] Forestier R, Françon A, Graber-Duvernay B. Les paramètres de validité d'un essai thérapeutique et leur influence sur l'élaboration d'une médecine fondée sur les preuves : revue de la littérature. Ann Réadapt Méd Phys 2005; 48(5): 250-8.

[8] Fremanian J. Validation des échelles d'évaluation en médecine physique et de réadaptation. Comment apprécier leurs propriétés psychométriques. Ann Réadapt Méd ¨Phys 2005; 48: 281-7.

[9] Sutton AJ, Duval SJ, Tweedie RL, Abrams KR, Jones DR. Empirical assessment of effect of publication bias on meta-analyses. BMJ 2000; 320: 1574-7.

[10] Balint GP, Buchanan WW, Adam A, *et al*. The effect of the thermal mineral water of Nagybaracska on patients with knee joint OA-a double blind study. Clin Rheumatol 2007; 26(6): 890-4.

[11] Nguyen M, Revel M, Dougados M. Prolonged effects of 3 week therapy in a spa resort on lumbar spine, knee and hip OA: follow up after six months. A randomized clinical trial. Br J Rheumatol 1997; 36(1): 77-81.

[12] Cantarini L, Leo G, Giannitti C, Cevenini G, Barberini P, Fioravanti A. Therapeutic effect of spa therapy and short wave therapy in knee OA: a randomized, single blind, controlled trial. Rheumatol Int. 2007; 27(6): 523-9.

[13] Evcik D, Kavuncu V, Yeter A, Yigit Ilktur. The efficacity of balneotherapy and mud pack therapy in patients with knee OA. Joint Bone Spine 2007; 74(1):60-5.

[14] Fioravanti A, Iacoponi F, Bellisai B, Cantarini L, Galeazzi M. Short- and Long-Term Effects of Spa Therapy in Knee OA. Am J Phys Med Rehabil 2010;89(2): 125-32.

[15] Forestier R. Magnitude and duration of the effect of two spa therapy courses on knee and hip OA: an open prospective study in 51 consecutive patients. Joint Bone Spine 2000; 67 (4): 296-304.

[16] Forestier R, Desfour H, Tessier JM, *et al*. Spa therapy in the treatment of knee OA, a large randomised multicentre trial. Ann Rheum Dis. 2010; 69(4): 660-5.

[17] Karagülle M, Karagülle MZ, Karagülle O, Dönmez A, Turan M. A 10-day course of SPA therapy is beneficial for people with severe knee OA. A 24-week randomised, controlled pilot study Clin Rheumatol 2007; 12: 2063-71.

[18] Kovacs I, Bender T. The therapeutic effect of Czerketszolo thermal water in OA of the knee: a double blind controlled follow up study. Rheumatol Int 2002; 21(6): 218-21.

[19] Obadasi E, Karagülle MZ, Karagülle Z, Turan M, Karagülle O. Comparison of two spa therapy regimens in patients with knee OA, an exploratory study. Phys Med Rehab Kuror 2002; 12: 337-41.

[20] Sherman G, Zeller L, Avriel A, Friger M, Harari M, Sukenik S. Intermittent balneotherapy at the Dead sea area for patients with knee OA. Isr Med Assoc J 2009; 11(2): 88-93.

[21] Sukenik S, Mayo A, Neumann L, Flusser D, Codish S, Abu-Shakra M. Balneotherapy at the Dead sea for knee OA. Isr Med Assoc J 1999; 1(2): 83-5.

[22] Szucs L, Ratko I, Lesko T, Szoor I, Genti G, Balint G. Double blind trial on the effectiveness of the puspokladany thermal water on arthrosis of the knee joint. J Royal Scoc Health 1989:7-9.

[23] Tishler M Rosenberg O, Levy O *et al*. The effect of balneotherapy on OA. Is an intermittent regimen effective? Eur J Intern Med 2004; 15(2): 93-96.

[24] Vaht M, Birkenfeldt R, Ubner M. An eva.luation of the effect of differing lengths of spa therapy upon patients with OA (OA). Complement Ther Clin Pract 2008; 14(1): 60-4.

[25] Wigler I, Elkayam O, Paran D, Yaron M. Spa therapy for gonarthrosis: a prospective study. Rheumatol Int 1995; 15: 65-8.

[26] Yurkturan M, Yurkturan M, Alp A, Nasicilar A, Bingol U, Altan L, Sardpere G. Balneotherapy and tap water in the treatment of knee OA. Rheumatol int 2006; 27: 19-27.

[27] Cochrane T, Davey RC, Matthes Edwards SM. Randomised controlled trial of the cost-effectiveness of water-based therapy for lower limb OA. Health Technol Assess 2005; 9(31): 1-114.

[28] Foley A, Hlabert J, Hewitt T, Crotty M. Does hydrotherapy improve strength and physical function in patients with OA - a randomised controlled trial comparing a gym based and a hydrotherapy based strengthening programme. Ann Rheum Dis 2003; 62(12):1162-7.

[29] Fransen M, Nairn L, Winstanley J, Lam P, Edmonds J. Physical activity for OA management: a randomized controlled clinical trial evaluating hydrotherapy or Tai Chi classes. Arthritis Rheum 2007; 57(3): 407-14.

[30] Green J, Mc Kenna F, Redfern EJ, Chamberlain MA. Home exercises are as effective as outpatient hydrotherapy for OA of the hip. Br J Rheumatol 1993; 32: 812-5.

[31] Hinman RS, Heywood SE, Day AR. Aquatic physical therapy for hip and knee OA: results of a single-blind randomized controlled trial. Phys Ther. 2007; 87(1): 32-43.

[32] Patrick DL, Ramsey SD, Spencer AC, Kinne S, Belza B, Topolski TD. Economic evaluation of aquatic exercise for persons with OA. Med Care 2001; 39(5): 413-24.

[33] Flusser D, Abu-Shakra M, Friger M, et al.Therapy With Mud Compresses for Knee OA Comparison of Natural Mud Preparations With Mineral-Depleted Mud. J Clin Rheumatol 2002; 8: 197-203.

[34] Lund H, Weile U, Christensen R, et al. A randomized controlled trial of aquatic and land-based exercise in patients with knee OA. J Rehabil Med 2008; 40(2): 137-44.

[35] Perlman AI, Sabina A, Williams AL, Njike VY, Katz DL. Massage therapy for OA of the knee: a randomized controlled trial. Arch Intern Med 2006; 166(22): 2533-8.

[36] Silva LE, Valim V, Pessanha AP, Oliveira LM, Myamoto S, Jones A, Natour J. Hydrotherapy versus conventional land-based exercise for the management of patients with OA of the knee: a randomized clinical trial. Phys Ther 2008; 88(1):12-21.

[37] Bellometti S, Gallotti C, Pacileo G, Rota A, Tenconi MT. Evaluation of outcomes in SPA-treated osteoarthrosic patients. J Prev Med Hyg 2007; 48(1):1-4.

[38] Cetin N, Aytar A, Atalay A, Akman MN. Comparing hot pack, short-wave diathermy, ultrasound, and TENS on isokinetic strength, pain, and functional status of women with osteoarthritic knees: a single-blind, randomized, controlled trial. Am J Phys Med Rehabil 2008; 87(6): 443-51.

[39] Flusser D, Abu-Shakra M, Friger M, Codish S, Sukenik S. Therapy with mud compresses for knee OA: comparison of natural mud preparations with mineral-depleted mud. J Clin Rheumatol 2002; 8(4): 197-203.

[40] Giaquinto S, Ciotola E, Dall'armi V, Margutti F. Hydrotherapy after total knee arthroplasty. A follow-up study. Arch Gerontol Geriatr 2010; 51(1): 59-63.

[41] Gill SD, McBurney H, Schulz DL. Land-based versus pool-based exercise for people awaiting joint replacement surgery of the hip or knee: results of a randomized controlled trial. Arch Phys Med Rehabil 2009; 90(3): 388-94.

[42] Harmer AR, Naylor JM, Crosbie J, Russell T. Land-based versus water-based rehabilitation following total knee replacement: a randomized, single-blind trial. Arthritis Rheum 2009; 61(2): 184-91.

[43] Mahboob N, Sousan K, Shirzad A, et al. The efficacy of a topical gel prepared using Lake Urmia mud in patients with knee OA. J Altern Complement Med 2009; 15(11):1239-42.

[44] Rahmann AE, Brauer SG, Nitz JC. A specific inpatient aquatic physiotherapy program improves strength after total hip or knee replacement surgery: a randomized controlled trial. Arch Phys Med Rehabil 2009; 90(5): 745-55.

[45] Seto H, Ikeda H, Hisaoka H, Kurosawa H. Effect of heat- and steam-generating sheet on daily activities of living in patients with OA of the knee: randomized prospective study. J Orthop Sci 2008; 13 (3): 187-91.

[46] Stener-Victorin E, Kruse-Smidje C, Jung K. Comparison between electro-acupuncture and hydrotherapy, both in combination with patient education and patient education alone, on the symptomatic treatment of OA of the hip. Clin J Pain 2004; 20(3):179-85.

[47] Wang TJ, Belza B, Elaine Thompson F, Whitney JD, Bennett K. Effects of aquatic exercise on flexibility, strength and aerobic fitness in adults with OA of the hip or knee. J Adv Nurs 2007; 57(2): 141-52.

[48] Zelen M. A new design for randomized clinical trial. N Engl J Med 1979;31(22):1242-5.

[49] Zelen M. Randomized consent design for clinical trial: an update. Stat Med 1990; 9(6) : 645-56

[50] Hrobjartsson A, Gotzche PC. Is the placebo powerless? An analysis of clinical trial comparing placebo with no treatment. N Engl J Med 2001; 344: 1594-602.

CHAPTER 7

Acupuncture and Osteoarthritis: Practices and Evidences

K. Sanchez, S. Poiraudeau and F. Rannou[*]

Service de Médecine Physique et de Réadaptation, Hôpital Cochin, AP-HP, Université Paris Descartes, INSERM, Institut Fédératif de Recherche sur le Handicap (IFR 25), 27 rue du Faubourg Saint-Jacques, 75679 Paris Cedex 14

Abstract: Acupuncture is recommended as a non-pharmacological treatment option for patients with knee and hip osteoarthritis (OA). Acupuncture is a Chinese philosophy which aims to restore the body to normal health. The explained mechanisms consider that acupuncture nociceptive pathways are essential for acupuncture analgesia, which is mediated by different endogenous neurotransmitters, such as enkephalin and dynorphin, and probably decreases the local inflammatory response *via* N-methyl-d-aspartate receptors. Acupuncture increases pain threshold gradually, with a peak effect at 20-40 min; a tolerance mediated by choleystokinin octapeptide could be observed if a prolonged period of acupuncture stimulation is performed. Immunocytochemistry and imaging studies indicate that both pain and acupuncture activate the hypothalamicpituitary-adrenocortical axis.

The literature review shows that clinical effects are small when acupuncture is compared with sham for treating OA patients; however, few if any other commonly used treatments for OA meet the threshold for clinically relevant benefits. On the other hand, acupuncture exceeds the thresholds for clinical relevance when compared with a waiting list control and with some other active treatment control, but the absence of sham treatment as a control suggests that benefits are primarily due to expectation or placebo effects.

Keywords: Osteoarthritis, acupuncture, pain.

1. INTRODUCTION

The most recent evidence-based treatment guidelines from the UK National Institutes of Clinical Excellence [1] and the Osteoarthritis Research Society International [2] suggest that OA treatment should be multidisciplinary, with nonpharmacological treatments such as education, aerobic and resistance exercises, and weight loss as the "cornerstone" [1] or "initial focus" [2] of patient management, and with consideration also given to pharmacological options such as acetaminophen when further treatment is required. In a systematic review of clinical guidelines performed by *Zhang et al.* [2], five of the eight guidelines considered acupuncture as an OA treatment modality. The guidelines subsequently developed by an international multidisciplinary group of experts using a Delphi process, recommended acupuncture as one of the 12 possible non-pharmacological modalities for treating OA. However, this recommendation achieved only a 69% consensus among the guideline committee members [2].

Acupuncture is considered as a Complementary and Alternative Medicine (CAM) therapy and patients with OA usually seek out CAM therapies [3-5]. The need for additional safe and effective treatments for OA is clear. Acupuncture is a safe treatment that has a low risk for serious side effects [6-7]. Therefore it is relevant to know if acupuncture is effective for treating OA.

The aim of this chapter is to describe the neurophysiological basis for acupuncture, and present the practice of and evidence for acupuncture treatment for patients with OA.

2. USE OF COMPLEMENTARY AND ALTERNATIVE MEDICINE

According to the 2002 National Health Interview Survey (N=30785), which included a section on CAM

*Address correspondence to F. Rannou: Service de Médecine Physique et de Réadaptation, Hôpital Cochin (AP-HP),Université Paris Descartes, 27 rue du Faubourg Saint-Jacques,75679 Paris Cedex 14, France; Tel: + 33 1 58 41 25 35; Fax: + 33 1 58 41 25 45; E-mail: francois.rannou@cch.aphp.fr

Yves Henrotin, Kim Bennell and Francois Rannou (Eds)

therapy, 41% of those who reported having chronic arthritis had used some form of CAM [5]. Of these, 24% used biologically based therapies, 21% used mind/body therapies, and 1.2% used acupuncture. Another survey found that 67% of people with OA in primary care clinics were currently using at least one type of CAM therapy [4], with glucosamine and chondroitin being by far the most commonly used therapies. All other CAM therapies for treating OA are used far less frequently than these drugs. For example, acupuncture is used by only 2% of patients for osteoarthritis [4].

3. ACUPUNCTURE

Acupuncture is an important part of health care in Asian culture that can be traced back almost 3000 years. This ancient Chinese intervention consists of applying pressure, needling, heat, and electrical stimulation to specific acupuncture points to restore patients to good health [8, 9].

In 1992, the American Congress established the Office of Alternative Medicine. Based upon the results of well-designed and appropriately controlled clinical trials, the National Institutes of Health (NIH), in November 1997, issued a statement that supported the efficacy of acupuncture for specific conditions, such as pain, nausea, and vomiting [10]. In 1998, acupuncture became the most popular CAM modality prescribed by western physicians [11]. In 1999 the National Center for Complementary and Alternative Medicine was established within the NIH.

3.1. Traditional Acupuncture Theory

Traditional Chinese acupuncture is a philosophy that focuses more on prevention than on treatment of illnesses. This philosophy presumes that there are two opposing and complementary forces that coexist in nature: Yin and Yang. These two forces interact to regulate the flow of "vital energy," known as Qi. When a person is in "good health," Yin and Yang are in balance, and the flow of Qi is smooth and regular. When Yin and Yang become "unbalanced," there are disturbances in Qi, which lead to illness and disease. The ancient Chinese believed that Qi flows through a network of channels called "meridians", which bring Qi from the internal organs to the skin surface. Along these meridians there are acupuncture points that can be stimulated to correct the imbalance and restore the body to normal health [8].

During an acupuncture session, the "De Qi" sensation is frequently described by patients as soreness, numbness, ache, fullness, or warm sensation that is achieved during manipulation of the acupuncture needles [8-9]. This sensation coincides with acupuncturists describing a feeling of the needle being caught as it is twirled (*e.g.*, the "fish took the bait" or "the needle is stuck to a magnet") [12]. Wang *et al.* [13] suggested that type II afferent fibers are responsible for the sensation of numbness, type III afferent fibers for fullness (heavy, mild aching), and type IV afferent fibers for soreness.

3.2. Modern Acupuncture Theory

The traditional Chinese perspective is not based on anatomical, physiological, or biochemical evidence, and thus cannot form the basis of a mechanistic understanding of acupuncture. Western theories are primarily based on the presumption that acupuncture induces signals in afferent nerves that modulate spinal signal transmission and pain perception in the brain. In 1976, Pomeranz proposed that acupuncture stimulation activates A-δ and C afferent fibers in muscle, causing signals to be transmitted to the spinal cord, which then results in a local release of dynorphin and enkephalins [14]. These afferent pathways propagate to the midbrain, triggering a sequence of excitatory and inhibitory mediators in the spinal cord. The resultant release of neurotransmitters, such as serotonin, dopamine, and norepinephrine onto the spinal cord leads to pre- and post-synaptic inhibition and suppression of the pain transmission. When these signals reach the hypothalamus and pituitary, they trigger the release of adrenocorticotropic hormones (ACTH) and endorphins. Pomeranz's theory was confirmed by a large series of experiments [15, 16].

3.3. Neurophysiologic Mechanisms (Table 1)

3.3.1. Volunteer Data

One of the first volunteer studies that examined the scientific basis of acupuncture analgesia was published in 1973 by a group of investigators who used a model of acute pain mediated by potassium iontophoresis with gradual increases of electrical current [17]. The volunteers were randomized to receive acupuncture at large intestine 4 (LI4) and stomach 36 (ST36) or intramuscular morphine. The investigators found that both acupuncture and morphine increased the subjects' pain threshold by an average of 80%–90%. The increasing of the pain threshold was gradual, with a peak effect at 20 – 40 min, followed by an exponential decay with a half-life of approximately 16 min, despite continued acupuncture stimulation. When researchers injected local anesthetic into these acupuncture points before the stimulation, the acupuncture became ineffective in increasing the pain threshold, suggesting that an intact sensory nervous system is essential for the transmission of acupuncture signals. Analgesic effects were the same regardless of which side of the body was stimulated. Finally, a greater cumulative effect was observed when multiple acupuncture points were stimulated simultaneously. In a follow-up study, Lim *et al.* [18] found that direct stimulation of peripheral nerve sensory fibers increased the pain threshold in a similar manner to that caused by standard acupuncture technique.

3.3.2. Experimental Data

The difficulty in developing suitable animal models has been one of the major obstacles in the experimental study of the mechanism of acupuncture anesthesia [19].

In 1973, Han and his colleagues [19] applied acupuncture to a rabbit for 30 min to achieve an analgesic effect. They then removed the cerebrospinal fluid and infused it into the lateral ventricle of an acupuncture-naïve recipient rabbit, resulting in an increase in the pain threshold in the recipient rabbit and suggesting that analgesia was associated with the release of neuromodulatory substances into the cerebrospinal fluid.

Table 1: Neurophysiologic mechanism.

	Intervention	Results
Volunteer Data	Acupuncture at LI4, ST36 vs. Intramuscular morphine [17]. Direct stimulation of peripheral nerve sensory fibers vs. Acupuncture [18].	Increase of subjects' pain threshold.
Experimental Data	Cerebral spinal fluid of a rabbit receiving acupuncture infused into the lateral ventricle of an acupuncture naïve recipient rabbit [19].	Increase of subjects' pain threshold.
	Opioid antagonist-naloxone injected in a mouse model [20, 21].	Block the acupuncture induced analgesic activity.
	Repeated EA stimulation to a rat model [22].	Decrease of the analgesic effect .
	Immersion of a rat footpad into 52°C water vs. Acupuncture stimulation (4Hz) in rats [23-25].	Activation of the hypothalamic-pituitary- adrenocortical axis.

Pomeraz and Chiu [14], using a mouse model, found that administration of the opioid antagonist-naloxone blocked the acupuncture-induced analgesic activity. Similar results were obtained in a human model [21].

When Electro Acupuncture (EA) stimulation was applied to a rat model for a 30-min period and repeated over six consecutive sessions, the analgesic effect diminished progressively [22]. This research confirmed the tolerance to acupuncture.

Pan *et al.* [23-25] studied whether there is an overlap of central pathways between noxious stimulation (caused by immersing the footpad into 52°C water) and acupuncture stimulation (4Hz) in rats. Their data suggested that both stimuli activate the hypothalamic-pituitary-adrenocortical axis analogous to stress, but with a specific activation of the mediobasal hypothalamic nuclei, and no activation of intermediate lobe. Furthermore, the authors confirmed the need of intact nociceptive primary afferent input to transmit both EA and noxious stimulation signals to the central nervous system.

3.4. Central Nervous System Imaging Studies

Advanced imaging technologies have been introduced, including Positron Emission Tomography (PET), Single-Proton Emission Computer Tomography (SPECT), and functional magnetic resonance imaging (fMRI). These powerful imaging technologies have made it possible to noninvasively visualize the anatomic and functional effects of acupuncture stimulation in the human brain.

3.4.1. PET Studies

Using PET imaging, Alavi *et al.* [26] observed that a group of patients who suffered from chronic pain also had asymmetry of the thalamus, which disappeared after acupuncture treatment. However, the study did not include a sham-control group.

Hsieh *et al.* [27] visualized the effect of De Qi sensation. They found that only acupuncture stimulation at LI4 (large intestine) with De Qi sensation activated the hypothalamus. Biella *et al.* [28] sequentially applied acupuncture and sham acupuncture at bilateral ST36 (stomach) and LU5 (lung) during a PET scanning sequence and showed that acupuncture, but not sham treatment, activated the left anterior cingulum, superior frontal gyrus, bilateral cerebellum, and insula, as well as the right medial and inferior frontal gyri. These are the same areas activated by acute and chronic pain [29]. This finding suggests a possible mechanism for acupuncture analgesia. Pariente *et al.* [30] thought that, in addition to the direct analgesic effect of acupuncture, the anticipation and belief of a patient might also affect the level of therapeutic outcome. Using PET image, investigators reported that both true and sham acupuncture activated the right dorsolateral prefrontal cortex, anterior cingulated cortex, and midbrain, and they suggested that these central nervous system areas are involved in nonspecific factors such as expectation. They also found that only true acupuncture caused a greater activation in insula ipsilateral to the site of stimulation, proposing that the insula region of the brain has a specific role in acupuncture analgesia.

3.4.2. SPECT Studies

Newberg *et al.* [31] used radioisotope hexamethylpropyleneamine oxime to image the brain of patients suffering from chronic pain and healthy volunteers without pain. The investigators found significant asymmetric uptake in the thalamic regions of patients with chronic pain, but not in the healthy control group, which reversed or normalized after 20–25 min of acupuncture stimulation, coinciding with the reduction of pain. Analogous findings in PET studies were reported [26].

3.4.3. fMRI Studies

a. Manual Acupuncture Stimulation

There are some discrepancies between Wu *et al.* [32] and Hiu *et al.* [33, 34], concerning the central nervous system areas activated during acupuncture. For Wu *et al.* [32], traditional acupuncture stimulation activates the hypothalamus and nucleus accumbens, but deactivates the rostral part of the anterior cingulate cortex, the amygdale formation, and the hippocampal complex. Minimal acupuncture activates the supplementary motor area and anterior cingulate cortex and frontal as well as parietal operculum. Superficial pricking activates the primary somatosensory cortex, the thalamus, and the anterior cingulate cortex. In contrast, Hui *et al.* [33, 34], found that subjects who experienced De Qi deactivated the frontal pole, ventromedial prefrontal cortex, cingulate cortex, hypothalamus, reticular formation, and the cerebellar vermis. Subjects who experienced pain instead of De Qi sensation activated the anterior cingular gyrus, caudate, putamen, and anterior thalamus. When these subjects experienced both De Qi and pain, the CNS responses were mixed with predominance of activation at the frontal pole, anterior, middle, and posterior cingulated.

These discrepancies between studies could be explained by differences in the duration of acupuncture stimulation (1 min vs. 2 min), the conscious perceptions of nociceptive input from acupuncture stimulation experienced by study subjects and the methodology of fMRI image analysis [35].

Ulett *et al.* [36] suggested that the periaqueductal gray (PAG) region is associated with perception and modulation of noxious stimuli during acupuncture. It was confirmed by Liu *et al.* [37].

b. EA Stimulation

To investigate the direct modulatory effects of EA stimulation in pain responses, Zhang *et al.* [38] studied a group of healthy volunteers using fMRI scanning during experimental cold pain with real or sham EA stimulation. Only the subjects who received EA reported a reduction of pain. The brain images showed an acupuncture-induced increased activation in the bilateral somatosensory area, medial prefrontal cortices and Brodmann area (BA32), and a decreased activation in the contralateral primary somatosensory areas BA7 and BA24 (anterior cingulated gyrus). With sham stimulation, there were no fMRI image changes. As these areas are frequently involved in pain stimulation, the authors concluded that EA induces analgesic effects *via* modulation of both the sensory and emotional aspects of pain processing. This study again demonstrates that the hypothalamus-limbic system plays an important role in acupuncture analgesia.

An fMRI study by Zhang *et al.* [39] found that the low-frequency (2 Hz) EA stimulations activated the contralateral primary motor area, supplementary motor area, and ipsilateral superior temporal gyrus, while deactivating the bilateral hippocampus. In contrast, high-frequency (100 Hz) EA stimulations activated the contralateral inferior parietal lobules, ipsilateral anterior cingulated cortex, nucleus accumbens and pons, while deactivating the contralateral amygdala. Therefore, low and high-frequency EA stimulation appear to be mediated by different brain networks and alternating high/low-frequency EA stimulations may provide the additional analgesia benefit by activating both systems simultaneously [40, 41].

c. Studies Comparing Different Acupuncture Stimulations

Napadow *et al.* [42] compared manual acupuncture, EA at 2 and 100 Hz, and tactile control stimulation at ST36 in a group of healthy volunteers. They reported that low-frequency EA produced more widespread fMRI signal changes than manual acupuncture stimulation. Both EA and manual acupuncture produced more widespread responses than simple tactile stimulation, and that although acupuncture stimulation activated the anterior insula, it deactivated the limbic and paralimbic structures that include the amygdala, anterior hippocampus, cortices of the subgenual and retrocingulate, ventromedial prefrontal cortex, and frontal and temporal lobes. EA at both high and low frequencies produced a significant signal increase in the anterior middle cingulated cortex. However, only low-frequency EA produced activation at the raphe area. Therefore, fMRI studies support the hypothesis that the limbic system is essential to acupuncture-induced analgesia despite the consequences of the specific modalities.

4. INTERNATIONAL RECOMMENDATIONS

The OARSI [2] and EULAR [43, 44] recommendations agree that the optimal management of knee and hip OA requires a combination of non-pharmacological and pharmacological treatment modalities.

Concerning the management of knee and hip OA, the 12th recommendation of OARSI 2008 [2], mentions that acupuncture may be of symptomatic benefit in patients with knee OA, with a Strength of Recommendation (SOR) of 59% (95% CI 47-71). Acupuncture is recommended as a modality of therapy for the symptomatic treatment of patients with knee or hip OA in 5/8 existing guidelines in which it was considered, and its recommendation achieved a 69% consensus following a Delphi exercise. A summary of the evidence for its clinical efficacy in lower limb joint OA which was available to the OARSI treatment guideline development group showed moderate effect size (ES) for pain (ES=0.51, 95% CI 0.23, 0.79), stiffness (ES=0.41, 95% CI 0.13, 0.69) and function (ES=0.51, 95% CI 0.23, 0.79) with a number needed to treat (NNT) of 4 (95% CI 3, 9) for clinically significant relief of pain. The last update of OARSI 2010 [45], considers that ES for relief of pain is lower when comparing acupuncture with sham acupuncture (ES=0.35, 95% CI 0.15, 0.55), it also diminishes with time (ES=0.13, 95% CI 0.01, 0.24, 6 months after treatment). Similar findings were observed with function.

Nevertheless, the EULAR evidence based recommendations for the management of hip [43] and knee [44] OA, does not take into account acupuncture therapy as one of the nonpharmacological options. For both, knee and hip OA, it recommends education, exercise, appliances (sticks, insoles) and weight reduction.

5. PRACTICE AND EVIDENCE

Current evidence from several high-quality RCTs suggests that acupuncture may be an effective treatment for older patients with OA. However, drawing general conclusions is complicated because the effects of acupuncture differ depending on whether acupuncture is compared with a waiting list, usual care, or sham control [46]. Table **2**.

Table 2: Acupuncture vs. sham, waiting list or other active treatment, and acupuncture plus another active treatment vs. other active treatment alone.

References	Design	Population	Intervention	Follow-up	Outcomes measured	Results
Berman *et al.* (1999)	RCT	73 patients with knee OA	- Acupuncture - Control : Waiting list	12 weeks	- WOMAC index - Lequesne scale	Significant improvement in WOMAC and Lequesne scales for the intervention group at 4 and 8 weeks after treatment.
Sangdee *et al.* (2002)	RCT	193 out-patients with knee OA	- Placebo - Diclofenac - EA - Diclofenac plus EA Paracetamol was the rescue analgesic during the study	4 weeks	- The amount of paracetamol taken/week - Visual analog scale (VAS) - Western Ontario and McMaster Universities (WOMAC) OA Index - Lequesne's functional index - 50 feet-walk time -The orthopedist's and patient's opinion of change	A significantly improvement in VAS between the EA and placebo group as well as the EA and diclofenac group. The improvement in Lequesne's functional index also differed significantly between the EA and placebo group. A significant improvement in WOMAC pain index between the combined and placebo group.
Vas *et al.* (2004)	RCT	97 outpatients presenting knee OA	- Acupuncture plus diclofenac (n = 48) -Placebo acupuncture plus diclofenac (n = 49).		-Intensity of pain (visual analogue scale) - Pain, stiffness, and physical function subscales of the WOMAC osteoarthritis index - Dosage of diclofenac taken during treatment - The profile of quality of life in the chronically ill (PQLC) instrument	- Acupuncture plus diclofenac is more effective than placebo acupuncture plus diclofenac taking into account the WOMAC index and the visual analogue scale. -Significant changes in physical capability (p = 0.021) and psychological functioning (p = 0.046) in the PQLC for the intervention group.
Berman *et al.* (2004)	RCT	570 patients with knee OA (mean age [±SD], 65.5 ± 8.4 years).	- 23 true acupuncture sessions - Controls received 6 two-hour sessions over 12 weeks or 23 sham acupuncture sessions over 26 weeks.	26 weeks	- Primary outcomes: Changes in the Western Ontario and McMaster Universities Osteoarthritis Index (WOMAC) pain and function scores at 8 and 26 weeks. - Secondary outcomes: patient global assessment, 6-minute walk distance, and physical health scores of the 36-Item Short-Form Health Survey (SF-36).	Acupuncture seems to provide improvement in function (mean difference, -2.5 [CI, -4.7 to -0.4]; P - 0.01), and pain relief (mean difference, -0.87 [CI,-1.58 to -0.16]; p= 0.003), as an adjunctive therapy for knee OA when compared with credible sham acupuncture and education control groups.
Tukmachi *et al.* (2004)	RCT	30 patients with knee OA	- Group A: acupuncture alone - Group B: acupuncture and symptomatic medication - Group C: symptomatic medication for the first 5 weeks and then had a course of acupuncture	1 month	- Visual analogue pain scale (VAS) - The Western Ontario McMaster (WOMAC)	- A highly significant improvement in pain (VAS) after the courses of acupuncture in groups A (p=0.012) and B (p=0.001); there was no change in group C until after the course of acupuncture, when the improvement was significant (p=0.001). - Similarly significant changes were seen with the WOMAC pain and stiffness scores.

Witt *et al.* (2005)	RCT	294 patients with chronic knee OA	-Acupuncture (n=150) -Minimal acupuncture (superficial needling at non-acupuncture points; n=76) -Waiting list control (n=74).	52 weeks	-WOMAC - A modified version of the German Society for the Study of Pain survey (Schmerzempfindungs-Skala [SES]) - Depression scale (Allgemeine Depressionsskala [ADS]) - The German version of the SF-36 - Sociodemographic characteristics, numerical rating scales for pain intensity, questions about workdays lost, and global assessments - Number of days with pain and medication	Acupuncture treatment had significant and clinically relevant short-term (effects after 8 weeks) when compared to minimal acupuncture or no acupuncture treatment in patients with knee OA.
Witt *et al.* (2006)	RCT with an additional nonrandomized arm	3,633 patients with chronic pain due to knee (mean ± SD age 61.8 ± 10.8 years)	- Acupuncture group (N=357) - Control group (N=355) - Nonrandomized acupuncture group (N=2,921) All patients received usual medical care	6 months	- WOMAC (pain, function) - Quality of life (SF-36)	Acupuncture plus routine care is associated with marked clinical improvement in patients with chronic OA–associated pain of the knee or hip, 3 and 6 moths after treatment. Changes in outcome in nonrandomized patients were comparable with those in randomized patients who received acupuncture.
Scharf *et al.* (2006)	RCT	1007 patients with chronic pain for at least 6 months due to knee OA	- 10 sessions of Traditional Chinese Acupuncture (TCA). - 10 sessions of sham acupuncture - 10 physician visits All patients received 6 physiotherapy sessions and as-needed anti-inflammatory drugs.	26 weeks	- WOMAC score -Secondary outcomes: SF-12 and global patient assessment	Compared with physiotherapy and as-needed anti-inflammatory drugs, addition of either TCA or sham acupuncture led to greater improvement in WOMAC score at 26 weeks. The absence of significant difference between TCA and sham acupuncture, suggest that the observed differences could be due to placebo effects, differences in intensity of provider contact, or a physiologic effect of needling regardless of whether it is done according to TCA principles.
Foster NE *et al.* (2007)	RCT	352 adults aged 50 or more with a clinical diagnosis of knee OA	- Advice and exercise (n=116) - Advice and exercise plus true acupuncture (n=117) -Advice and exercise plus non-penetrating acupuncture (n=119).	Six months	- Primary outcome: change in scores on the Western Ontario and McMaster Universities osteoarthritis index pain subscale at six months. -Secondary outcomes: function, pain intensity, and unpleasantness of pain at two weeks, six weeks, six months, and 12 months.	- The addition of acupuncture to a course of advice and exercise for knee OA provided no additional improvement in pain scores. - Small benefits in pain intensity and unpleasantness were observed in both acupuncture groups.

| Williamson et al. (2007) | RCT | 181 patients awaiting knee arthroplasty | - Acupuncture for 6 weeks
- Physiotherapy for 6 week
- Standardized advice | 3 months | - Main outcome measure: Oxford Knee Score questionnaire (OKS) (primary)
-Secondary outcomes: WOMAC, pain visual analogue scale, Hospital Anxiety and Depression Score (HAD), 50m timed walk, and duration of hospital stay following knee arthroplasty. | Authors demonstrated that patients with severe knee osteoarthritis can achieve a short-term reduction in OKS when treated with acupuncture. |

5.1. Acupuncture Versus Sham

The recent Cochrane review by Manheimer *et al.* [47], considering 9 RCTs, found that acupuncture at short-and long-term improves knee or hip OA pain (standardized mean difference -0.28, 95% confidence interval -0.45 to -0.11, 9 trials, 1835 participants; I^2 64%), function (-0.28, -0.46 to -0.09; 9 trials, 1829 participants, I^2 69%), and symptom severity (-0.29, -0.50 to -0.09, 9 trials, 1767 participants, I^2 74%), compared with sham control, but the results are heterogeneous.

For the two RCTs that found clinically relevant benefits of acupuncture, the credibility of the sham was not tested and the informed consent procedure was not described. Sangdee *et al.* [48] used patch electrodes attached to the acupuncture knee points with mock electrical stimulation as sham acupuncture, and Vas *et al.* [49], sham needles which did not penetrate the skin, leading to limitations in blinding. Nevertheless, despite this bias, the acupuncture benefits could be explained by the use of intensive electrical stimulation at the acupuncture points, which likely produce stronger analgesics effects [36]. Two other large sham RCTs [50-51] used fully needle penetrating shams in similar points to true acupuncture and the effects were compared with a non acupuncture group. Benefits of sham acupuncture suggest that the sham points were probably physiologically active and inappropriate as controls. This is explained by the Diffuse Noxious Inhibitory Control (DNIC) mechanism, which suggests that noxious stimuli (needles in this case) applied to any part of the body can produce analgesic effects, even at distant sites [52, 53]. Another bias was a positive attitude towards acupuncture and high expectations of a benefit in participants. Foster *et al.* [54] used non penetrating sham acupuncture at the same true acupuncture points leading a highly credible and believable sham. However the benefits of this therapy suggest that these sham needles may have some physiological activity due to a massaging effect on the acupuncture points.

5.2. Acupuncture Versus Waiting List

When Manheimer *et al.* [47] analyzed 4 RCTs comparing acupuncture with a waiting list control, acupuncture was associated with greater clinically relevant short term improvements in knee or hip OA pain (0.96, -1.19 to -0.72; 4 trials; 884 participants; $I^2 = 41$%), function (-0.89, -1.18 to -0.60; 3 trials; 864 participants; $I^2 = 64$%) and symptom severity (-0.92, -1.16 to -0.67; 3 trials; 864 participants; $I^2 = 52$%).

5.3. Acupuncture Versus Other Active Treatment

The literature is controversial when acupuncture is compared with other active treatments. When Berman *et al.* [55] compared acupuncture to supervised OA education control and Scharf *et al.* [51], to a physician consultation control (with a physiotherapy co-intervention), they found that acupuncture was associated with short-and long-term improvements in pain and function. Conversely, Williamson *et al.* [56] showed no differences between acupuncture and home exercises/advice leaflet nor supervised exercise.

Manheimer *et al.* [47] mention that the major limitation of these two last designs (acupuncture vs. waiting list or another active treatment) is the lack of blinding. Therefore the clinically relevant benefits of acupuncture in comparison to a waiting list or to an active treatment control might be partly explained by either non-specific effect associated with the patient-acupuncturist relationship [57, 58] or to expectations of a benefit by participants [59].

5.4. Acupuncture Plus Another Active Treatment Versus other Active Treatment Alone

There is only one clinical trial in which acupuncture has been evaluated as an additive treatment. Foster *et al.* [54] found that there was no greater improvements when using acupuncture as an adjuvant to a physiotherapy program (including a supervised home exercise) than a physiotherapy program alone.

5.5. Safety Considerations in the Use of Acupuncture

In a systematic review of the English literature of adverse effects of acupuncture for any condition from 22 countries between 1965 and 1999, Lao [60] found a total of 202 case reports, half of which were from the United States. The most common complications were infections and internal organ and tissue injuries. Eighty percent of the infections reported (94 cases) were hepatitis. However, since 1988, there were no new cases of hepatitis, and only 8 cases of infections of any type associated with acupuncture. This may reflect the introduction of US certification requirements for clean needle techniques and the use of disposable needles, which are required by law in most states. Even less frequent were internal organ and tissue injuries—60 cases over the 35 years [61].

In the most recent revision [47] eight RCTs describing adverse events found similar frequency between the acupuncture and control groups. No serious adverse events associated with acupuncture were reported; minor bruising and bleeding at needle insertion sites ranged from 0% [56, 62-64] to 45% [48]. This wide variation is explained by the sparse reporting and no definitive definition of what constitutes a side effect of acupuncture and what is considered an inherent part of treatment.

It appears that the risks from acupuncture are minimal when acupuncturists are licensed, use disposable needles, and practice clean needle techniques. However, patients should inform their acupuncturist if they are taking anticoagulant medication or have a cardiac pacemaker [65-66].

5.6. Acupoints Used in OA Therapy

5.6.1. For Knee OA

Acupuncture points include: ST34 (stomach), ST35, ST36, LIV8 (liver), SP9 (spleen), SP10, GB34 (gallbladder), KI6 (kidney), SJ5 (San Jiao), LI4 (large intestine), TH5 (triple heater meridian), SP6, LIV3, ST44, KI3, BI60, GB41 [50, 54]. Extra points: Xijan, Heding [50].

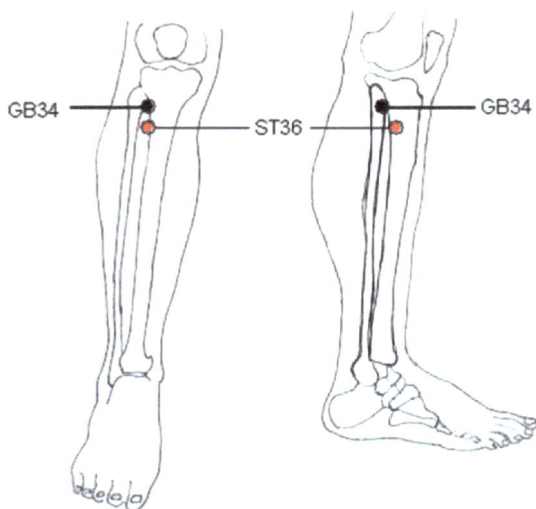

Figure 1: Location of acupoints, GB34 and ST36 [35].

5.6.2. For Hip OA

Acupuncture points include: GB29, GB30, GB31, GB34, GB43, ST44, LI4 [50].

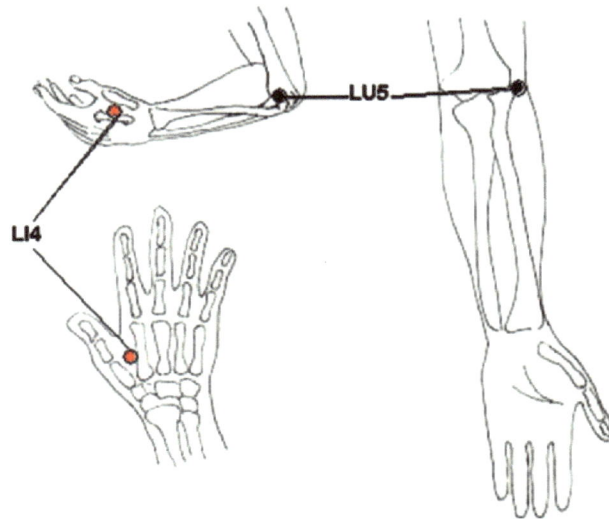

Figure 2: Location of acupoint, LI4 [35].

6. COSTS

In addition to efficacy and safety, patients and clinicians also need to take into account costs because acupuncture treatment often needs to be paid at least in part, by patients. Witt *et al.* [67], found that the cost per QALY (quality-adjusted life year) of acupuncture in comparison with sham acupuncture was about $30, 519.

CONCLUDING REMARKS

Acupuncture therapy is recommended by OARSI as an option in the non pharmacological OA treatment [2]. No serious adverse effects are associated with its application [48, 56, 62-64].

When acupuncture is compared with sham, the effects are small; however, few if any other commonly used treatments for OA meet the threshold for clinically relevant benefits [68]; for example NSAIDs which are used by half of all people with painful OA, also do not meet this threshold [69]. These small effects of individual therapies could be interpreted as a need for a multidisciplinary approach to OA management, combining several non-pharmacological therapies [43]. On the other hand, acupuncture exceeds the thresholds for clinical relevance, when compared with a waiting list control and some other active treatment control, but the absence of sham treatments as controls suggests that the benefits are mainly due to expectation or placebo effects.

Consequently, for future trials, researchers [47] suggest that (i) monthly acupuncture treatments are maintained in the months prior to a long term assessment, due to the fact that benefits may attenuate over time once treatment is ceased [55, 70]; (ii) the use of an electrical stimulation over needles is evaluated, (iii) an adequate number of treatments is investigated, (iv) the preferences and expectations (before and after the intervention) and the potential effects of pre treatment preferences on study outcomes to elicit a placebo effect or a meaning response are assessed; (v) participants are not told that acupuncture is one of the treatments being investigated (this could be in the form of a Zelen trial); and (vi) a non-insertive sham is used with a credibility test before and during the trial.

It is necessary to include cost-effectiveness analysis in trials evaluating acupuncture in all types of peripheral joint OA. Lastly, combinative treatment with and without acupuncture procedures are needed in order to assess the weight of the acupuncture effect in multiple treatment modalities of OA as generally occurs in clinical practice.

REFERENCES

[1]   National Collaborating Centre for Chronic Conditions. Osteoarthritis: national clinical guideline for care and management in adults. London: Royal College of Physicians, 2008.

[2]   Zhang W, Moskowitz RW, Nuki G, et al. OARSI recommendations for the management of hip and knee osteoarthritis, Part II: OARSI evidence-based, expert consensus guidelines. Osteoarthritis Cartilage 2008; 16: 137-162.

[3]   Rao JK, Mihaliak K, Kroenke K, Bradley J, Tierney WM, Weinberger M. Use of complementary therapies for arthritis among patients of rheumatologists. Annals of internal medicine 1999; 131 (6):409-16.

[4]   Herman CJ, Allen P, Hunt WC, Prasad A, Brady TJ. Use of complementary therapies among primary care clinic patients with arthritis. Prev Chronic Dis 2004; 1: A12.

[5]   Quandt SA, Chen H, Grzywacz JG, Bell RA, Lang W, Arcury TA. Use of complementary and alternative medicine by persons with arthritis: results of the National Health Interview Survey. Arthritis Rheum 2005; 53: 748-755.

[6]   Cherkin DC, Sherman KJ, Deyo RA, Shekelle PG. A review of the evidence for the effectiveness, safety, and cost of acupuncture, massage therapy, and spinal manipulation for back pain. Ann Intern Med 2003; 138: 898-906.

[7]   Melchart D, Weidenhammer W, Streng A, *et al*. Prospective investigation of adverse effects of acupuncture in 97,733 patients. Arch Intern Med 2004; 164: 104-5.

[8]   Liu G, Akira H. Basic principle of TCM. In: Liu G, Akira H, eds. Fundamentals of acupuncture and moxibustion. Tianjin, China: Tianjin Science and Technology Translation and Publishing Corporation 1994.

[9]   Pomeranz B. Scientific basis of acupuncture. In: Stux G, Pomeranz B, eds. Basis of acupuncture. 4th ed. Heidelberg: Springer-Verlag 1998.

[10]   NIH consensus developmental panel on acupuncture. JAMA 1998; 280: 1518-24.

[11]   Astin JA, Marie A, Pelletier KR, Hansen E, Haskell WL. A review of the incorporation of complementary and alternative medicine by mainstream physicians. Arch Intern Med 1998; 158: 2303-10.

[12]   Langevin HM, Churchill DL, Fox JR, Badger GJ, Garra BS, Krag MH. Biomechanical response to acupuncture needling in humans. J Appl Physiol 2001; 91: 2471-8.

[13]   Wang K, Yao S, Xian Y, Hou Z. A study on the receptive field on acupoints and the relationship between characteristics of needle sensation and groups of afferent fibres. Sci Sin 1985; 28: 963-71.

[14]   Pomeranz B, Chiu D. Naloxone blockade of acupuncture analgesia: endorphin implicated. Life Sci 1976; 19: 1757-62.

[15]   Cheng RSS, Pomeranz B. Monoaminergic mechanism of electroacupuncture analgesia. Brain Res 1981; 215: 77-92.

[16]   Cheng RS, Pomeranz B. Electroacupuncture analgesia is mediate by sterospecific opiate receptors and is reversed by antagonists of type I receptors. Life Sci 1980; 26: 631-8.

[17]   Research Group of Acupuncture Anesthesia PMC. The effect of acupuncture on human skin pain threshold. Chin Med J 1973; 3: 151-7.

[18]   Lim T, Loh T, Kranz H, Scott D. Acupuncture-effect on normal subjects. Med J Aust 1977; 1: 440-2.

[19]   Research Group of Acupuncture Anesthesia PMC. The role of some neurotransmitters of brain in finger acupuncture analgesia. Sci Sin 1974; 117: 112-30.

[20]   Sjolund BH, Ericksson M. Increased cerebrospinal fluid levels of endorphins after electroacupuncture. Acta Physiol Scand 1977; 100: 382-4.

[21]   Mayer DJ. Antagonism of acupuncture analgesia in man by the narcotic antagonist naloxone. Brain Res 1977; 121: 368-72.

[22]   Han JS, Tang J. Tolerance to electroacupuncture and its cross tolerance to morphine. Neuropharmacology 1981; 20: 593-6.

[23]   Pan B, Castro-Lopes J, Coimbra A. Activation of anterior lobe corticotrophs by electroacupuncture or noxious stimulation in the anaesthetized rat, as shown by colocalization of Fos protein with ACTH and beta-endorphin and increased hormone release. Brain Res Bull 1996; 40: 175-82.

[24]   Pan B, Castro-Lopes J, Coimbra A. C-fos expression in the hypothalamo-pituitary system induced by electroacupuncture or noxious stimulation. Neuroreport 1994; 5: 1649-52.

[25]   Pan B, Castro-Lopes J, Coimbra A. Chemical sensory deafferentation abolishes hypothalamic pituitary activation induced by noxious stimulation or electroacupuncture but only decreases that caused by immobilization stress. A c-fos study. Neuroscience 1997; 78: 1059-68.

[26]   Alavi A, LaRiccia P, Sadek Ah, Newberg AS, Lee L, Teich H, Lattanand C, Mozley PD. Neuroimaging of acupuncture in patients with chronic pain. J Altern Complement Med 1997; 3: S41-53.

[27]   Hsieh JC, Tu CH, Chen FP, Chen MC, Yeh TC, Cheng HC, W YT, Liu RS, Ho LT. Activation of the hypothalamus characterizes the acupuncture stimulation at the analgesic point in human: a positron emission tomography study. Neurosci Lett 2001; 307: 105-8.

[28]   Biella G, Sotgiu ML, Pellegata G, Paulesu E, Castiglioni I, Fazio F. Acupuncture produces central activations in pain regions. Neuroimage 2001; 14: 60-6.

[29]   Casey K, Minoshima S, Morrow T, Koeppe R. Comparison of human cerebral activation pattern during cutaneous warmth, heat pain, and deep cold pain. J Neurophysiol 1996; 76: 571-81.

[30]   Pariente J, White P, Frackowiak RSJ, Lewith G. Expectancy and belief modulate the neuronal substrates of pain treated by acupuncture. Neuroimage 2005; 25: 1161-7.

[31]   Newberg AB, Lariccia PJ, Lee BY, Farrar JT, Lee L, Alavi A. Cerebral blood flow effects of pain and acupuncture: a preliminary single-photon emission computed tomography imaging study. J Neuroimaging 2005; 15: 43-9.

[32]   Wu MT, Hsieh JC, Xiong J, *et al.* Central nervous pathway for acupuncture stimulation: localization of processing with functional MR imaging of the brain preliminary experience. Radiology 1999; 212: 133-41.

[33]   Hui KKS, Liu J, Makris N, *et al.* Acupuncture modulates the limbic system and subcortical gray structures of the human brain: evidence from fMRI studies in normal subjects. Hum Brain Mapp 2000; 9: 13-25.

[34]   Hui KKS, Liu J, Marina O, *et al.* The integrated response of the human cerebro-cerebellar and limbic systems to acupuncture stimulation at ST 36 as evidenced by fMRI. Neuroimage 2005; 27: 479-96.

[35]   Wang S-M, Kain ZN, White P. Acupuncture analgesia I: The scientific basis. Pain Med 2008; 106: 602-10.

[36]   Ulett GA, Han S, Han JS. Electroacupuncture: mechanisms and clinical application. Biol Psychiatry 1998; 44: 129-38.

[37]   Liu WC, Feldman SC, Cook DB, Hung DL, Xu T, Kalnin AJ, Komisaruk BR. fMRI study of acupuncture-induced periaqueductal gray activity in humans. Neuroreport 2004; 15: 1937-40.

[38]   Zhang W, Jin Z, Huang J, Ahang YW, Luo F, Chen AC, Han JS. Modulation of cold pain in human brain by electric acupoint stimulation: evidence from fMRI. Neuroreport 2003; 14: 1591-6.

[39]   Zhang WT, Jin Z, Cui GH, *et al.* Relations between brain network activation and analgesic effect induced by low vs. high frequency electrical acupoint stimulation in different subjects: a functional magnetic resonance imaging study. Brain Res 2003; 982: 168-78.

[40]   Hamza MA, White PF, Ahmend HE, Ghoname ES. Effect of the frequency of transcutaneous electrical nerve stimulation on the postoperative opioid analgesic requirement and recovery profile. Anesthesiology 1999; 91: 1232-8.

[41]   Wang Y, Zhang Y, Wang W, Cao Y, Han JS. Effects of synchronous or ashynchronous electroacupuncture stimulation with low versus high frequency on spinal opioid release and tail flick nociception. Exp Neurol 2005; 192: 156-62.

[42]   Napadow V, Makris N, Liu J, Kettner NW, Kwong KK, Hui KK. Effects of electroacupuncture versus manual acupuncture on the human brain as measured by fMRI. Hum Brain Mapp 2005; 24: 193-205.

[43]   Jordan KM, Arden NK, Doherty M, *et al.* EULAR Recommendations 2003: an evidence based approach to the management of knee osteoarthritis: Report of a Task Force of the Standing Committee for International Clinical Studies Including Therapeutic Trials (ESCISIT). Ann Rheum Dis 2003; 62(12):1145-55.

[44]   Zhang W, Doherty M, Peat G *et al.* EULAR evidence based recommendations for the management of hip osteoarthritis: report of a task force of the EULAR Standing Committee for International Clinical Studies Including Therapeutics (ESCISIT). Ann Rheum Dis 2005; 64: 669-681.

[45]   Zhang W, Nuki G, Moskowitz RW, *et al.* OARSI recommendations for the management of hip and knee osteoarthritis . Part III: changes in evidence following systematic cumulative update of research published through January 2009. Osteoarthritis Cartilage 2010; 18: 476-99.

[46]   Manheimer E, Linde K, Lao L, Bouter LM, Berman, BM. Meta-analysis: Acupuncture for Osteoarthritis of the Knee. Ann Intern Med 2007; 146: 868-877.

[47]   Manheimer E, Cheng K, Linde K, *et al.* Acupuncture for peripheral joint osteoarthritis. Cochrane Database Syst Rev 2010; (1): CD001977.

[48]   Sangdee C, Teekachunhatean S, Sananpanich K, *et al.* Electroacupuncture versus diclofenac in symptomatic treatment of osteoarthritis of the knee: a randomized controlled trial. BMC Compl Altern Med 2002; 2: 3.

[49]   Vas J, Mendez C, Perea-Milla E, *et al.* Acupuncture as a complementary therapy to the pharmacological treatment of osteoarthritis of the knee: randomised controlled trial. BMJ 2004; 329(7476): 1216.

[50] Witt CM, Jena S, Brinkhaus B, Liecker B, Wegscheider K, Willich SN. Acupuncture in patients with osteoarthritis of the knee or hip: a randomized, controlled trial with an additional nonrandomized arm. Arthritis Rheum 2006; 54(11): 3485-93.

[51] Scharf HP, Mansmann U, Streitberger K, *et al.* Acupuncture and knee osteoarthritis: a three-armed randomized trial. Ann Int Med 2006; 145(1): 12-20.

[52] Le Bars D, Dickenson AH, Besson JM. Diffuse noxious inhibitory controls (DNIC). I. Effects on dorsal horn convergent neurones in the rat. Pain 1979; 6(3): 283-304.

[53] Lewith GT, Machin D. On the evaluation of the clinical effects of acupuncture. Pain 1983; 16(2):111-27.

[54] Foster NE, Thomas E, Barlas P, *et al.* Acupuncture as an adjunct to exercise based physiotherapy for osteoarthritis of the knee: randomised controlled trial. BMJ 2007; 335: 436.

[55] Berman BM, Lao L, Langenberg P, Lee WL, Gilpin AM, Hochberg MC. Effectiveness of acupuncture as adjunctive therapy in osteoarthritis of the knee: a randomized, controlled trial. Ann Int Med 2004; 141(12): 901-10.

[56] Williamson L, Wyatt MR, Yein K, Melton JT. Severe knee osteoarthritis: a randomized controlled trial of acupuncture, physiotherapy (supervised exercise) and standard management for patients awaiting knee replacement. Rheumatology (Oxford) 2007; 46(9):1445-9.

[57] Paterson C, Dieppe P. Characteristic and incidental (placebo) effects in complex interventions such as acupuncture. BMJ 2005; 330(7501):1202-5.

[58] Kaptchuk TJ, Kelley JM, Conboy LA, *et al.* Components of placebo effect: randomised controlled trial in patients with irritable bowel syndrome. BMJ 2008; 336(7651): 999-1003.

[59] Linde K, Witt CM, Streng A, Weidenhammer W, Wagenpfeil S, Brinkhaus B, *et al.* The impact of patient expectations on outcomes in four randomized controlled trials of acupuncture in patients with chronic pain. Pain 2007; 3: 264-71.

[60] Lao L. Safety issues in acupuncture. J Altern Complement Med. 1996; 2: 27-31.

[61] Berman B. A 60-year-old woman considering acupuncture for knee pain. JAMA 2007; 297: 1697-705.

[62] Berman BM, Singh BB, Lao L, *et al.* A randomized trial of acupuncture as an adjunctive therapy for osteoarthritis of the knee. Rheumatology (Oxford) 1999; 38: 346-54.

[63] Fink MG, Wipperman B, Gehrke A. Non-specific effects of traditional Chinese acupuncture in osteoarthritis of the hip. Complement Therap Med 2001; 9(2): 82-9.

[64] Haslam R. A comparison of acupuncture with advice and exercises on the symptomatic treatment of osteoarthritis of the hip-a randomised controlled trial. Acupunct Med 2001; 19(1):19-26.

[65] Ernst E, White AR. Prospective studies of the safety of acupuncture: a systematic review. Am J Med 2001; 110: 481-485.

[66] MacPherson H, Thomas K, Walters S, Fitter M. The York acupuncture safety study: prospective survey of 34 000 treatments by traditional acupuncturists. BMJ 2001; 323: 486-487.

[67] Witt C, Selim D, Reinhold T, *et al.* Cost effectiveness of acupuncture in patients with headache, low back pain and osteoarthritis of the hip and the knee. In: 12th annual symposium on complementary health care - abstracts: 19th-21st September 2005, Exeter, UK; Focus on Altern Complement Ther 2005; 10: 57-8.

[68] Bjordal JM, Klovning A, Ljunggren AE, Slordal L. Short-term efficacy of pharmacotherapeutic interventions in osteoarthritic knee pain: A meta-analysis of randomised placebo-controlled trials. Eur J Pain 2007; 11(2):125-38.

[69] Bjordal JM, Ljunggren AE, Klovning A, Slordal L. Non-steroidal anti-inflammatory drugs, including cyclo-oxygenase-2 inhibitors, in osteoarthritis knee pain: meta-analysis of randomized placebo controlled trials. BMJ 2004; 329: 1317-22.

[70] Witt C, Brinkhaus B, Jena S, *et al.* Acupuncture in patients with osteoarthritis of the knee: a randomized trial. Lancet 2005; 366: 136-43.

CHAPTER 8

Bracing for Osteoarthritis

J. Beaudreuil[*]

Service de Rhumatologie, Hôpital Lariboisière, AP-HP, Université Paris 7, Paris, France

Abstract: Bracing for osteoarthritis (OA) involves the use of splints, tape, sleeves, and unloading knee braces. It is part of recommended non-pharmacological treatment for osteoarthritis of the thumb base and knee. Randomized clinical trials back these recommendations. Evidence that splints improve pain and disability in patients with thumb base OA is now provided. Weaker evidence appears for knee bracing including taping, sleeves and unloading braces. Low rate of adherence and safety issues should also be considered before using current unloading knee braces for knee OA. If bracing is to be used, a health professional should check to ensure the suitability of the device and provide patient education. Patient education includes knowledge of the aims of treatment, and encouragement to contact the therapist if they feel that the splint needs adjustment, or if they have any side effect or questions.

Keywords: Brace, tape, insole, splints, osteoarthritis.

1. INTRODUCTION

Bracing involves the use of a spectrum of external devices including splints, tape, sleeves, and unloading knee braces. Bracing is part of recommended non-pharmacological treatments for osteoarthritis (OA) of the thumb base and knee [1-3]. Randomized clinical trials and reviews now provide useful information for an evidence-based analysis of their effectiveness and their safety, in these indications. Physicians interested in OA should be aware of this emerging literature, including the advantages and disadvantages of bracing for OA in daily practice. When using bracing at any site, a health professional should check to ensure the suitability of the device. Patients using bracing should also be educated. Patient education includes knowledge of the aims of treatment, and encouragement to contact the therapist if they feel that the brace needs adjustment, if pain increases while wearing the brace, or if they have side effects such as skin erosion. It might be important to emphasise that a brace should not be used as a stand-alone treatment but should complement other treatment options. Also, the decision to use a brace should be based on whether the patient demonstrates improvement on subjective and objective outcomes, particularly as individual responses vary.

2. BRACING FOR THUMB BASE OA

2.1. Description of Bracing for Thumb Base OA

Devices for thumb base OA aim to immobilize the carpometacarpal joint and the opening of the first web if it is reduced by the disease. In practice, they are semi-rigid and rigid splints that can be either prefabricated or custom-made by health professionals. Splints systematically cover the carpometacarpal joint and the thenar eminence (Fig. 1). Crossing the metacarpophalangeal joint or the wrist has been proposed too.

2.2. Effectiveness of Bracing for Thumb Base Osteoarthritis

Effectiveness of splinting for thumb base OA has recently been investigated in a high-powered multicenter randomized clinical trial with non splint parallel comparison [4] (Table 1). One hundred twelve patients with thumb base OA were included. Half were asked to wear a custom-made rigid splint during the night. The splint covered the carpo-metacarpal joint, the thenar eminence and the metacarpal joint, but not the wrist. Patients were assessed at 1 and 12 months. Treatment adherence was high since 93% of patients

*Address correspondence to J. Beaudreuil: Service de Rhumatologie,Hôpital Lariboisière, AP-HP, Université Paris 7, Paris, France; E-mail : johann.beaudreuil@lrb.aphp.fr

Yves Henrotin, Kim Bennell and Francois Rannou (Eds)

reported wearing the splint 5 to 7 nights a week at 1 month and 86% at 12 months. No adverse event directly attributable to the splint was reported. At 1 month no between-group difference was observed. However, wearing a splint significantly improved pain and disability at 12 months. Two small crossover trials compared a short splint covering the carpometacarpal joint only with a long splint covering the carpometacarpal and the metacarpal joints, in thumb base OA [5, 6]. They individually provided conflicting short-term results, but pooled analysis indicated more pain relief from the long splint than from the short one [2]. Two other low-powered trials compared either two splints and exercise regimens either elastic, elastic semi-rigid and nonelastic semi-rigid orthoses [7, 8]. They found no relevant difference at short-term follow-up.

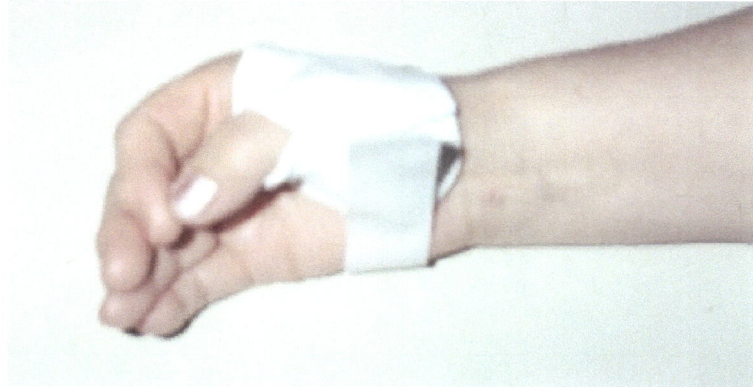

Figure 1: Splint for thumb base OA. Custom-made device crossing the carpomatacarpal joint and the metacarpal joint.

Wearing a splint for thumb base OA appears therefore to reduce pain and disability as compared with nonsplint control. Studies also suggest higher effectiveness with a long splint than with a short one. Taken together these data back the recommendation of bracing for thumb base OA.

3. BRACING FOR KNEE OA

3.1. Description of Bracing for Knee OA

Bracing for knee OA includes the use of rest orthoses, tape, sleeves and unloading braces [9-11]. Rest orthoses are comprised of a stiff composite and aim to immobilize the joint without providing any dynamic, corrective or functional effect. Tape, sleeves and unloading braces are functional devices. Knee taping for OA involves the application of adhesive rigid strapping tape to the patella with the aim of centering the patella within the trochlear grove [12] and decreasing the loads applied to the lateral part of the patellofemoral joint. The tape can also be applied with the aim of reducing load on soft tissues structures around the knee such as the infrapatellar fat pad.

Table 1: Randomized trials for thumb base osteoarthritis.

References	Design	Population	Intervention	Follow-up	Outcome	Results
Buurke *et al.* 1999 [7]	controlled, crossover, randomized	n = 10	- elastic device - elastic semi-rigid splint - semi-rigid splint		Pain, pinch force, disability	- No inter-group difference
Weiss *et al.* 2000 [5]	controlled, crossover, randomized	n = 26	- short splint - long splint	1 week	CMC subluxation, pain, pinch force, disability, satisfaction, patient preference	- Short splint > long splint: Patient preference

Weiss *et al.* 2004 [6]	controlled, crossover, randomized	n = 25	- short splint - long splint	1 week	CMC subluxation, pain, pinch force, disability, satisfaction, patient preference	- Long splint > short splint: Pain, pinch force, patient preference - Short splint > long splint: CMC subluxation
Wajon *et al.* 2005 [8]	controlled, parallel, randomized	n = 40	- strap plint and abduction exercises - short-oppenens splint and pinch exercises	6 weeks	Pain, pinch force, disability	- No inter-group difference
Rannou *et al.* 2009 [4]	controlled, parallel, randomized	n = 112	- splint - no splint	12 months	Pain, pinch force, thumb mobility, disability, OA progression, co-interventions	- Splint > no splint: Pain and disability

CMC: carpometacarpal. OA: osteoarthritis.

Some of the knee sleeves are elastic nonadhesive orthoses aimed at realigning the patella or providing frontal femorotibial stabilisation (Fig. **2**). Unloading braces are composed of external stems, hinges and straps. They aim to decrease compressive loads transmitted to the joint surfaces, either in the medial or lateral femorotibial compartment, depending on the valgus or varus position of the device. As with splints for thumb base OA, unloading braces can be prefabricated or custom-made by health professionals.

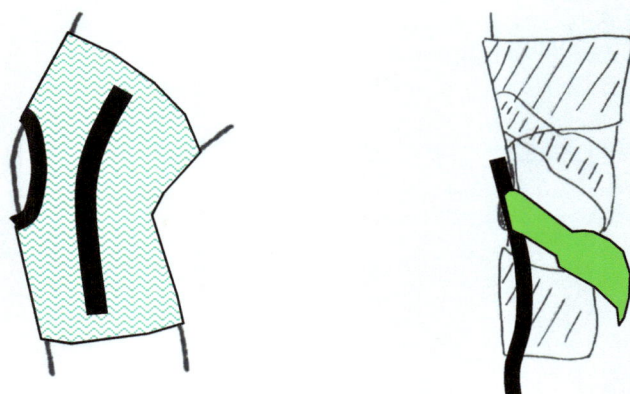

Figure 2: Bracing for knee osteoarthritis. Left: knee sleeve with peripatellar and lateral devices. Right: unloading knee brace.

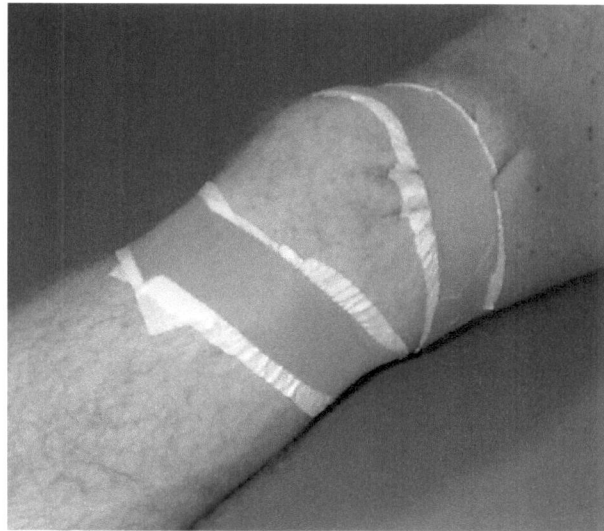

Figure 3: Knee tape designed to realign the patella and unload the infrapatellar fat pad.

3.2. Effectiveness of Bracing for Knee OA

Investigation of clinical daily practice in French physiatrists and rheumatologists has indicated a low rate of prescription of bracing for knee OA [9, 10]. Recommendations and recent randomized clinical trials suggest however that some types of bracing could be useful in patients with knee osteoarthritis.

3.2.1. Effectiveness of Rest Orthoses

The effectiveness of rest orthoses for knee OA has not been studied in clinical trials [10] with only descriptive reviews suggesting their usefulness. Rest orthoses could be used for transient immobilization in times of acute pain flares or increased knee effusion. However, this hypothesis needs to be tested in clinical trials.

3.2.2. Effectiveness of Knee Taping

Effectiveness of taping for knee osteoarthritis has been investigated in 5 clinical randomized trials [9, 13-17] (Table **2**). Three were controlled parallel-group trials [9, 15, 17] and two were crossover trials [13, 16]. In these studies, patients had femorotibial OA with or without patellofemoral involvement (Fig. **3**). None of the patients was withdrawn because of side effects. A randomized controlled parallel-group trial compared the use of three weeks of taping with sham taping and no intervention [15]. Taping induced a significant reduction in pain as compared with sham and no intervention at three weeks. The pain relief persisted three weeks after tape removal as compared with no intervention only. The other controlled parallel-group trial compared a program including taping and physical exercises with sham ultrasound therapy and failed to detect any between-group difference [17]. Crossover studies reinforced the idea of short-term pain reduction with knee taping as compared with sham or no taping, in patients with knee OA [13, 16]. They also indicated short-term superiority of medial taping, pulling the patella medially, and loose bandage, as compared with lateral taping and standard-sized bandage respectively [13,14].

Table 2: Randomized trials for Knee osteoarthritis.

References	Design	Population	Intervention	Follow-up	Outcome	Results
			Knee tape			
Cushnaghan *et al.* 1994 [12]	controlled, crossover, randomized	n = 14, femorotibial and patellofemoral OA	- medial taping of the patella - lateral taping - neutral taping	4 days	Pain, global assessment	- Medial taping > lateral and neutral taping: Pain and global assessment

Hassan *et al.* 2002 [13]	controlled, crossover, randomized	n = 68, femorotibial OA ± patellofemoral OA	- loose bandage - standard-sized bandage - no bandage	1 day	Pain, proprioception, postural sway	- Loose bandage > no bandage: Pain and postural sway
Hinman *et al.* 2003 [14]	controlled, parallel, randomized	n = 87, femorotibial OA ± patellofemoral OA	- taping above and below the patella - sham tape - no tape	3 weeks	Pain, WOMAC, SF-36	- Taping > sham and no tape: Pain - Taping > no tape: Disability
Hinman *et al.* 2003 [15]	controlled, crossover, randomized	n = 18, femorotibial OA ± patellofemoral OA	- taping above and below the patella - sham tape - no tape	1 day	Pain, observed disability	Taping > sham and no tape: Pain
Bennell *et al.* 2005 [16]	controlled, parallel, randomized	n = 140, knee OA	- taping above and below the patella plus physiotherapy - sham physiotherapy	12 weeks	Pain, WOMAC, SF-36	- No inter-group difference
			Knee sleeves			
Berry *et al.* 1992 [18]	controlled, parallel, randomized	n = 170, knee OA	- sleeve - no sleeve	6 weeks	Pain, global assessment	- Sleeve > no sleeve: Pain and gobal improvement
Kirkley *et al.* 1999 [17]	controlled, parallel, randomized	n = 119, medial femoro-tibial OA	- unloader-brace - neoprene sleeve - no bracing	6 months	WOMAC, MACTAR, observed disability	- Unloader-brace > sleeve: Pain and observed disability - Unloader-brace > no bracing: Pain and disability Sleeve > no bracing: Pain and stiffness
Mazzuca *et al.* 2004 [19]	controlled, parallel, randomized	n = 52, knee OA	- heat-retaining sleeve standard - sleeve	4 weeks	WOMAC	No inter-group difference
			Unloading knee braces			
Horlick *et al.* 1993 [21]	controlled, cross over, randomized	n = 39, medial femoro-tibial OA	- unloader-brace - neutral brace - no brace	6 weeks	Femoro-tibial angle, pain and disability	- Unloader-brace > no brace: Pain
Kirkley *et al.* 1999 [17]	controlled, parallel, randomized	n = 119, medial femoro-tibial OA	- unloader-brace - neoprene sleeve - bracing (40)	6 months	WOMAC, MACTAR, observed disability	- Unloader-brace > sleeve: Pain and observed disability - Unloader-brace > no bracing: Pain and disability Sleeve > no bracing: Pain and stiffness
Self *et al.* 2000 [23]	controlled, cross over, randomized	n = 5, medial femoro-tibial OA	- unloader-brace - no brace	1 day	Adductor moment	- Unloader brace > no brace: Adductor moment
Birmingham *et al.* 2001 [24]	controlled, cross over, randomized	n = 20, genu varum with OA	- unloader-brace - no brace	1 day	Proprioception, postural control	- Unloader brace > no brace: Proprioception
Richards *et al.* 2005 [25]	controlled, cross over, randomized	n = 12, genu varum with OA	- unloader-brace - simple hinged brace - no brace	6 months	Walk analysis, pain and disability	- Unloader and simple hinged braces > no brace: Peak force at stance and propulsive peak force - Unloader brace > no brace: Disability
Brouwer *et al.* 2006 [26]	controlled, parallel, randomized	n = 117, medial or lateral knee OA	- unloader-brace - no brace	12 months	Pain, disability	- Unloader-brace > no brace: Pain and disabilty

| Draganich *et al.* 2006 [20] | controlled, cross over, randomized | n = 10, genu varum with OA | - custom-made unloader-brace
- off-the-shelf unloader-brace
- no brace | 4 weeks | Femorotibial angle, adductor moment, WOMAC | - Custom-made and off-the-shelf braces > no braces:
Pain and stiffness
- Custom-made > off-the-shelf braces and no braces:
Femorotibial angle, adductor moment and disability |
| Van Raaij *et al.* 2010 [22] | controlled, parallel, randomized | n = 91, medial knee OA | - unloader-brace
- laterally wedged insole | 6 months | Femorotibial angle, pain WOMAC | - No inter-group difference |

OA: osteoarthritis. WOMAC = Western Ontario MC Master, MACTAR = MacMaster Toronto Arthritis questionnaire.

Taping appears therefore well tolerated in patients with knee OA. Even if not exclusively tested in those with patellofemoral involvement, and despite some conflicting results, knee taping seems to be useful in providing a short-term improvement in pain as compared with sham or no taping intervention. Furthermore, data suggest that medial taping is more effective than lateral taping.

Skin care is important to minimise the risk of adverse effects especially when tape is applied to older skin. Patients should initially be screened to ensure they are appropriate for taping and caution should be exercised with individuals with a history of skin conditions or allergies to adhesive tapes or bandages. Hypoallergenic undertape should always be used in all patients to protect skin from direct contact by the rigid strapping tape that is used to realign the patellar and unload soft tissues. The majority of skin damage is caused by frequent removal of tape. Thus in older patients with knee OA, tape should be removed and re-applied less frequently than in younger people. Patients should be instructed to carefully remove the tape in a slow and controlled manner so as to minimise risk of skin damage. In the case of skin irritation, tape should be removed and the skin rested from taping until the damage has healed. Ongoing taping may not be appropriate for some patients.

In clinical practice, patients are usually taught by the therapist how to tape their knee themselves, thus allowing taping to be used at home as a self-management strategy for relief of knee pain. However, it is not known whether self-taping is as effective as therapist-applied tape as this has not been researched specifically to date.

3.2.3. Effectiveness of Knee Sleeves

Effectiveness of knee sleeves for knee OA has been investigated in three randomized controlled parallel-group trials [18-20] (Table **2**). Simple neoprene knee sleeves decreased pain at 6-month follow-up as compared with no sleeve treatment [17]. Sleeves with a silicon peripatellar device have also been compared with no sleeve treatment [18]. They decreased pain and induced subjective improvement after 6-week follow-up. Finally, heat-retaining sleeves composed of lycra, polyester and aluminium fibers have been compared with standard devices [19]. There was no difference in pain, stiffness and physical disability after four weeks of use. Therefore, clinical actions of knee sleeves do not appear to depend on any local thermal effect.

3.2.4. Effectiveness of Unloading Knee Braces

Randomized trials concerning unloading knee braces for knee osteoarthritis OA are more numerous than other types of braces (Table **2**). Most are low-powered crossover studies performed in patients with medial femorotibial OA. Their outcomes can be divided into biomechanical/sensorimotor and clinical results.

a. Biomechanical/Sensorimotor Results

The biomechanical effect of unloading knee braces have been assessed according to two criteria in randomized trials: 1) femorotibial angle and 2) adductor moment that serves as an indirect measure of medial femorotibial compartment loading during walking. Data concerning femorotibial angle are conflicting. One crossover trial showed a valgus effect with custom-made patient-adjustable unloading knee braces as compared with baseline values or with those of off-the-shelf unloading devices [21]. Two other studies failed to demonstrate any valgus effect [21, 22]. Adductor moment has been assessed in two crossover trials [21, 24]. Both indicated that custom-made unloading valgus knee braces decrease the adductor moment by a mean of 10-13% as compared with baseline values. This was not observed however, with off-the-shelf unloading braces [21].

In people with medial compartment knee OA who have frontal plane knee laxity and mediolateral instability, there is increased muscle activity and co-activation of antagonistic muscles [25-28]. While these muscle activation patterns may stabilise the knee, they can also increase joint reaction forces and exacerbate cartilage degeneration. A small cross-over study in 16 people with medial compartment knee OA and varus malalignment found that a brace either set at neutral alignment or at 4o valgus reduced muscle co-contraction [29].

One crossover trial indicated that valgus knee braces improved the ability to replicate knee joint position, as a proprioception marker [24]. However the mean difference between the braced and unbraced conditions was only 0.7°, which renders the clinical significance of these findings questionable. There was no effect on postural control in static position in this study. One other study showed an increase in peak force at stance and in vertical propulsive peak force with bracing as compared with baseline values [30]. However these results were observed with braces in the valgus or neutral position, without difference between the two positions.

b. Clinical Results

Six studies have evaluated the effect of unloading valgus knee bracing on pain and disability [18, 21-23, 29, 31] and support the effectiveness of such devices as compared with no bracing. The follow-up periods ranged from 6 weeks to 1 year. Furthermore, two trials showed better results with custom-made braces than with off-the-shelf braces or neoprene knee sleeves [18, 21]. One other indicated similar effect of unloading knee braces and laterally wedged insoles [23].

Data concerning adherence and safety have also been recorded. Discomfort and low rate of observance have been reported in patients using unloading knee braces [11, 12, 23, 31]. The main complaints were skin irritation and bad brace fit [23, 31]. The most serious were thromboembolic events [11, 12].

Finally, results of randomized trials suggest that unloading knee braces decrease the adductor moment and should be consequently able to reduce medial femorotibial compartment loading. The adductor moment during gait is one of only a few factors known to predict knee OA structural disease progression in humans [32]. Given the reduction in the adductor moment with knee braces, these have the potential to slow disease progression although this has not been directly evaluated. There is also clinical trial evidence for a beneficial effect of unloading knee braces on pain and disability in patients with medial femorotibial osteoarthritis. It is likely that the response to bracing varies in different subgroups of patients. This requires further investigation as it will assist clinicians in deciding which patients may be most appropriate for a trial of bracing therapy. However, the major remaining concerns with the current unloading knee braces are discomfort and low rate of adherence with potential side effects of which physicians and patients should be aware.

4. CONCLUDING REMARKS

Bracing is a useful adjunct in the treatment of patients with thumb base and knee osteoarthritis. There is evidence of the effectiveness of splints in patients with thumb base osteoarthritis from one high-powered study and other smaller trials. There is weaker evidence available for the effectiveness of knee bracing including taping, sleeves and unloading braces. Low rate of adherence and safety issues are also to be considered before using current unloading knee braces for knee osteoarthritis.

REFERENCES

[1]   Jordan KM, Arden NK, Doherty M, *et al.*EULAR Recommendations 2003: an evidence based approach to the management of knee osteoarthritis: Report of a Task Force of the Standing Committee for International Clinical Studies Including Therapeutic Trials (ESCISIT). Ann Rheum Dis 2003; 62 : 1145-1155.

[2]   Zhang W, Doherty M, Leeb BF, *et al.* EULAR evidence based recommendations for the management of hand osteoarthritis: report of a task force of EULAR Standing Committee for International Clinical Studies Including Therapeutics (ESCISIT). Ann Rheum Dis 2007; 66: 377-388.

[3]   Zhang W, Moskowitz RW, Nuki G, *et al.* OARSI recommendations for the management of hip and knee osteoarthritis, Part II: OARSI evidence-based, expert consensus guidelines. Osteoarthritis Cartilage 2008; 16: 137-162.

[4]   Rannou F, Dimet J, Boutron I, *et al.* Splint for base-of-thumb osteoarthritis. A randomized trial. Ann Intern Med 2009; 150: 661-669.

[5]   Weiss S, Lastayo P, Mills A, Bramlet D. Prospective analysis of splinting the first carpometacarpal joint: an objective, subjective, and radiographic assessment. J Hand Ther 2000; 13:218-226.

[6]   Weiss S, Lastayo P, Mills A, Bramlet D. Splinting the degenerative basal joint: custom-made or prefabricated neoprene? J Hand Ther 2004; 17: 401-406.

[7]   Buurke JH, Grady JH, de Vries J, Baten CT. Usability of thenar eminence orthoses: report of a comparative study. Clin Rehabil 1999; 13: 288-294.

[8]   Wajon A, Ada L. No difference between two splint and exercise regimens for people with osteoarthritis of the thumb: a randomized controlled trial. Aust J Physiother 2005; 51: 245-249.

[9]   Richette P, Sautreuil P, Coudeyre E, *et al.* Usefulness of taping in lower limb osteoarthritis. French clinical practice guidelines. Joint Bone Spine 2008; 75: 475-478.

[10]   Beaudreuil J, Bendaya S, Faucher M, *et al.* Clinical practice guidelines for rest orthosis, knee sleeves, and unloading knee braces in knee osteoarthritis. Joint Bone Spine 2009; 76: 629-636.

[11]   Rannou F, Poiraudeau S, Beaudreuil J. Role of bracing in the management of knee osteoarthritis. Curr Opin Rheumatol 2010; 22: 218-222.

[12]   Crossley KM, Marino GP, Macilquham MD, Schache AG, Hinman RS. Can patellar tape reduce the patellar malalignment and pain associated with patellofemoral osteoarthritis? Arthritis Rheum 2009; 61(12): 1719-25.

[13]   Cushnaghan J, McCarthy C, Dieppe P. Taping the patella medially: a new treatment for osteoarthritis of the knee joint? BMJ 1994; 308: 753-755.

[14]   Hassan BS, Mockett S, Doherty M. Influence of elastic bandage on knee pain, proprioception, and postural sway in subjects with knee osteoarthritis. Ann Rheum Dis 2002; 61: 24-28.

[15]   Hinmann RS, Crossley KM, McConnell J, *et al.* Efficacy of knee tape in the management of osteoarthritis of the knee: blinded randomised controlled trial. BMJ 2003; 327: 135.

[16]   Hinman RS, Crossley KM, McConnell J, *et al.* Immediate effects of adhesive tape on pain and disability in individuals with knee osteoarthritis. Rheumatology 2003; 42: 865-869.

[17]   Bennell KL, Hinman RS, Metcalf BR, *et al.* Efficacy of physiotherapy management of knee joint osteoarthritis: a randomized, double blind, placebo controlled trial. Ann Rheum Dis 2005; 64: 906-612.

[18]   Kirkley A, Webster-Bogaert S, Litchfield R, *et al.* The effect of bracing on varus gonarthrosis. J Bone Joint Surg 1999; 81-A: 539-548.

[19]   Berry H, Black C, Fernandes L, Bernstein RM, Whittington J. Controlled trial of a knee support (Genutrain) in patients with osteoarthritis of the knee. Eur J Rheumatol Inflamm 1992; 12: 30-34.

[20]   Mazzuca SA, Page MC, Meldrum RD, Brandt KD, Petty-Saphon S. Pilot study of the effects of a heat-retaining knee sleeve on joint pain, stiffness, and function in patients with knee osteoarthritis. Arthritis Rheum 2004; 51: 716-721.

[21]   Draganich L, Reider B, Rimington T, Piotrowski G, Mallik K, Nasson S. The effectiveness of self-adjustable custom and off-the-shelf bracing in the treatment of varus gonarthrosis. J Bone Joint Surg 2006; 88-A: 2645-2652.

[22]   Horlick SG, Loomer RL. Valgus knee bracing for medial gonarthrosis. Clin J Sport Med 1993; 3: 251-255.

[23]   Raaij TM, Reijman M, Brouwer RW, Bierma-Zeinstra SMA, Verhaar JAN. Medial knee osteoarthritis treated by insoles or braces. A randomized trial. Clin Orthop Relat Res 2010; 468:1921-1932.

[24]   Self BP, Greenwald RM, Pflaster DS. A biomechanical analysis of a medial unloading brace for osteoarthritis in the knee. Arthritis Care Res 2000; 13: 191-197.

[25]   Childs J, Sparto P, Fitzgerald G, Bizzini M, Irrgang J. Alterations in lower extremity movement and muscle activation patterns in individuals with knee osteoarthritis. Clinical Biomechanics 2004; 19:44-49.

[26]   Lewek M, Rudolph K, Snyder-Mackler L. Control of frontal plane laxity during gait in patients with medial compartment knee osteoarthritis. Osteoarthritis Cartilage 2004; 12: 745-751.

[27]   Lewek M, Ramsey D, Snyder-Mackler L, Rudolph K. Knee stabilization in patients with medial compartment knee osteoarthritis. Arthritis & Rheumatism 2005; 52: 2845-2853.

[28]   Ramsey DK, Briem K, Axe MJ, Snyder-Mackler L. A mechanical theory for the effectiveness of bracing for medial compartment osteoarthritis of the knee. J Bone Joint Surg Am 2007; 89(11): 2398-407.

[29]   Birmingham TB, Kramer JF, Kirkley A, Inglis JT, Spaulding SJ, Vandervoort AA. Knee bracing for medial compartment osteoarthritis: effects on proprioception and postural control. Rheumatology 2001; 40: 285-289.

[30]   Richards JD, Sanchez-Ballester J, Jones RK, Darke N, Livingstone BN. A comparison of knee braces during walking for the treatment of osteoarthritis of the medial compartment of the knee. J Bone Joint Surg 2005; 87-B: 937-939.

[31]   Brouwer RW, van Raaij TM, Verhaar JA, Coene LN, Bierma-Zeinstra SM. Brace treatment for osteoarthritis of the knee: a prospective randomized multi-centre trial. Osteoarthritis Cartilage 2006; 14: 777-783.

[32]   Miyazaki T, Wada M, Kawahara H, Sato M, Baba H, Shimada S. Dynamic load at baseline can predict radiographic disease progression in medial compartment knee osteoarthritis.Ann Rheum Dis. 2002; 61(7): 617-22.

CHAPTER 9

Insoles and Footwear in the Management of Knee Osteoarthritis

R.S. Hinman[*] and K.L. Bennell

Centre for Health, Exercise and Sports Medicine, Department of Physiotherapy, The University of Melbourne, Victoria, Australia.

Abstract: This chapter will review relevant research surrounding the use of insoles and footwear for knee osteoarthritis (OA). In particular, concepts relevant to the clinical application of these treatment techniques will be discussed. This chapter will examine the effects of common insole and footwear types on knee load, OA symptoms and disease progression. Increased joint loading increases the risk of OA progression, but is amenable to change. Given the prevalence of medial compartment OA, insoles and footwear largely aim to reduce the knee adduction moment, an indicator of medial compartment load. Lateral wedged insoles can reduce this moment but do not appear, at present, to slow disease progression. Whilst non- and quasi-experimental studies report favourable effects of lateral wedges on symptoms, most clinical trials have not been confirmatory. Medial wedged insoles show promise in relieving symptoms of lateral compartment disease. Walking in shoes increases joint load compared to barefeet. Shoes with a flat or low heel and that are flexible rather than stabilising in nature may be optimal for patients with knee OA, however effects of off-the-shelf shoes on OA symptoms are unknown. Promising shoe modifications currently under development include shoes that promote foot mobility and those with variable-stiffness or laterally wedged soles. In summary, insoles and footwear offer great potential as simple, inexpensive treatment strategies for knee OA. Further research is needed to evaluate their efficacy, particularly regarding their effects on knee symptoms and structural disease progression, and to determine which patient subgroups are most responsive.

Keywords: Osteoarthritis, insoles, footwear.

1. INTRODUCTION

Contemporary management of osteoarthritis (OA) aims not only to improve symptoms of disease, but also to reduce the risk of structural deterioration over time. Research over the past decade has highlighted the critical role that biomechanical factors, such as increased joint loading, play in onset and progression of OA. Most research has focussed on the knee joint, the most common lower limb site of OA. As such, the knee adduction moment is now widely accepted as an indicator of medial knee compartment load and offers a potential target for treatment strategies to slow disease course over time. Recent years have seen the development and implementation of various insole and footwear options specifically designed for reducing knee joint load, with the ultimate aim of alleviating knee pain and potentially slowing knee OA progression. This chapter will provide an overview of current insole and footwear treatment options for knee OA. Recent research findings will be discussed, including their clinical application.

2. EFFECT OF INSOLES ON KNEE LOAD, OA SYMPTOMS AND DISEASE PROGRESSION

Of the variety of shoe insoles available commercially for the management of musculoskeletal conditions, wedged insoles and medial arch supports are the most relevant for people with knee OA. Lateral wedged insoles, in particular, have been the most extensively researched and thus will be a major focus of this chapter.

2.1. Biomechanical Effects of Lateral Wedged Insoles

Lateral wedged insoles (Fig. **1**) were first proposed in the 1980's for knee OA [1, 2]. By virtue of the lower limb's closed kinetic chain during weightbearing, wedged insoles inserted into the shoes, or worn attached

---

*Address correspondence to R.S. Hinman: Centre for Health, Exercise and Sports Medicine, Department of Physiotherapy, The University of Melbourne, Parkville, Victoria, 3010; Tel: +61 3 8344 3223; Fax: +61 3 8344 4188; E-mail: ranash@unimelb.edu.au

Yves Henrotin, Kim Bennell and Francois Rannou (Eds)

to the barefoot *via* strapping or sock supports, can modify knee joint moments, particularly in the frontal plane. Due to their effects on frontal plane knee moments, lateral wedges are advocated for medial compartment OA and medial wedges for lateral compartment disease. Due to the predominance of medial tibiofemoral OA [3], lateral wedges have been the most widely researched.

Most, although not all, biomechanical research shows that lateral wedges reduce the adduction moment during walking by 4-12% (compared with barefoot or shoes alone) in people with medial knee OA [4-10]. It appears that lateral wedges exert a mechanical effect on the lower limb and cause a small lateral shift in the centre of pressure location of the ground reaction force [7, 8]. This likely decreases the knee joint moment arm, thereby reducing the knee adduction moment. Support for this hypothesis comes from mechanical modelling which has shown that as little as a 1mm lateral displacement of the centre of pressure decreases the knee adduction moment by 2% and results in a 1% reduction in medial knee compartment load [11]. As the majority of biomechanical research has evaluated only immediate effects of wearing lateral wedged insoles, it is not clear what effects the insoles have over the longer-term. Although only reported in abstract form, some research suggests that long-term use of lateral wedges may induce natural beneficial gait adaptations (reduced knee adduction moments when walking without wedges) [12]. However, similar adaptations were also evident with neutrally wedged insoles so it is unclear whether these changes are due to the insoles themselves, or natural history.

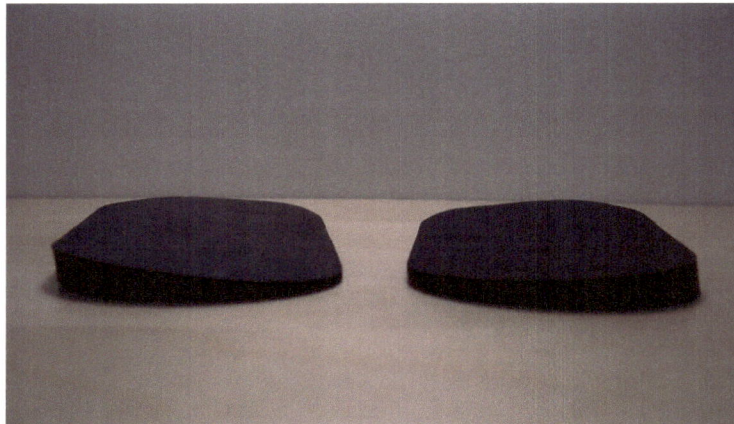

Figure 1: A typical pair of lateral wedged insoles. Note these insoles are wedged along the full length of the foot and are inclined approximately 5°.

The effects of lateral wedges on the knee adduction moment are not systematic, and research shows that biomechanical responses to lateral wedges vary across individuals. Although most studies report mean reductions in the knee adduction moment with lateral wedges, evaluation of individual responses shows that some people actually demonstrate an increased adduction moment with wedges [4-8, 13]. These findings suggest that patient and/or shoe characteristics may mediate biomechanical wedge effects and that certain patient subgroups may be more likely to respond. Disease severity may be important, with wedge-related decreases in the adduction moment observed in participants with mild but not moderate or severe OA [10]. Other characteristics that could mediate biomechanical responsiveness include forefoot and rearfoot alignment and motion, frontal plane alignment and baseline knee adduction moment. Of these, only rearfoot motion has been evaluated, with an abstract describing greater reductions in the adduction moment in participants with more frontal plane rearfoot motion [14]. Further studies in this area would help target lateral wedges to the most appropriate patient subgroups. It is also highly likely that shoe type mediates the biomechanical effects of lateral wedges but this has not been investigated specifically to date. Toda & Tsukimura [15] have, however, evaluated the influence of footwear in mediating the effect of lateral wedges on symptoms, and found that symptomatic effects are optimized when lateral wedges are worn with socks or flat footwear in comparison to shoes with heels. This is not surprising, given that heeled footwear is typically associated with an elevation in the knee adduction moment. This will be discussed in more detail later in this chapter.

Biomechanical effects are also influenced by specific design features of the wedged insole itself. For example, reductions in the knee adduction moment are directly related to the degree of wedging utilised, with greater wedging resulting in greater reductions in the knee adduction moment. However, from a clinical perspective it is important to consider that greater inclination of the lateral wedge (eg 10°) is more likely to cause foot discomfort [8]. Wedging may be standardized (using a predetermined amount, typically 5°), or customized to the individual. Whilst most research has investigated standardized lateral wedges, biomechanical benefits have been demonstrated also with a customized wedge (determined according to the minimal amount needed for maximal pain reduction during a lateral step-down) [4]. As no study has directly compared customized lateral wedges to standardized wedges, it is unclear if customization offers superior biomechanical benefits. We have shown that insoles wedged laterally along the full-length of the foot reduce the knee adduction moment more than an insole wedged at the rearfoot only [5]. This data supports prescription of full-length rather than rearfoot wedges. Finally, a combined treatment approach that uses elastic subtalar strapping with lateral wedges may reduce the adduction moment more than wedged insoles alone, particularly in patients with mild and moderate medial knee OA [9]. This may be because strapping causes valgus angulation of the talus leading to correction of the femorotibial angle, further reducing medial joint load [16].

Despite the potential for lateral wedged insoles to have adverse effects on other joints of the lower limb kinetic chain, or the contralateral limb, little research has evaluated the biomechanical effects of these insoles at sites other than the affected knee. Limited data suggest that lateral wedged insoles increase the peak eversion, eversion excursion and peak eversion moment at the foot with no effect at the hip [7, 17]. These findings suggest that health professionals should thoroughly screen a patient's foot before recommending lateral wedged insoles. Given that increased muscle torques will be required to control the excessive rearfoot eversion associated with wedges, such an insole could potentially aggravate individuals with foot pathology.

2.2. Symptomatic Effects of Lateral Wedged Insoles

Lateral wedged insoles are recommended for managing knee OA by almost all clinical guidelines [18]. However, results from non- and quasi-experimental studies, which generally show beneficial effects of lateral wedges on pain in knee OA [1, 6, 19-22], have not been confirmed by most randomised controlled trials conducted to date (Table **1**). One found that customized lateral wedges worn for 2 years significantly reduced the intake of non-steroidal anti-inflammatory drugs compared to neutral insoles, which may indicate a beneficial effect of lateral wedges. However pain, stiffness and function were similar between the wedged group and the control group at study completion [23, 24]. Similarly, a double-blind crossover trial found no statistical or clinical effect of a 5° lateral wedge worn for 6 weeks when compared to a flat neutral wedged insole [25], and a single-blind trial evaluating customised lateral wedges did not demonstrate beneficial effects over control insoles after 1 year [26]. In quasi-randomised studies of women with medial knee OA, lateral wedges combined with subtalar strapping provided better clinical benefit when compared to conventional wedges inserted into the shoes [16, 27-29]. However, several disadvantages of the combined intervention include more adverse effects [30] and the need for shoes larger than normal [29], which may limit the clinical applicability of this treatment approach. A clinical trial comparing different types of lateral wedges (a traditional insole inserted into shoes, an insole combined with subtalar strapping and an insole worn with a sock-type ankle supporter) and different types of footwear (flat shoes, socks, and heeled footwear) found that the strapped insole resulted in symptomatic improvement when worn with or without shoes, whilst the traditional inserted wedge was only beneficial if used in conjunction with socks or flat shoes [15]. Given that all of the trials failing to show a symptomatic effect of lateral wedges have not incorporated subtalar strapping and most have ignored the type of shoe worn in conjunction with the insole, it is possible that the sub-optimal choice of insole and shoe may have contributed to their non-significant findings.

In light of the individual variations in biomechanical response reported in the literature, it is also probable that not all patients with medial knee OA will benefit clinically from treatment with lateral wedged insoles. Better outcomes are observed in patients with less severe disease [1, 6, 20, 21, 25] and with increased lower limb lean mass [31], and in younger [31] and less obese [25] patients. We also found that individuals who experienced the greatest immediate reductions in pain and knee adduction moment with insoles demonstrated the greatest improvement in function after 3 months use [6]. Variation in daily usage of wedged insoles may also influence clinical outcome with a quasi-randomised trial suggesting that the greatest clinical benefits are achieved with 5-10 hours of daily use compared with <5 hours or >10 hours [32].

2.3. Structural Effects of Lateral Wedged Insoles

Given their effectiveness at reducing the adduction moment, lateral wedges have potential for slowing knee OA progression. However, in a randomised controlled trial, rearfoot lat- eral wedges had no effect on joint space narrowing rate over 2 years [24]. In a quasi-randomised trial comparing lateral wedges and subtalar strapping with conventional insertedwedges, no differences in progression rates were noted, although no control group was included [29]. These null findings may in part be due to the relative insensitivity of x-rays, to the wedge designs or to the heterogenous patient samples utilised. Whilst one study has reported that lateral wedged insoles delayed progression of joint space narrowing in medial knee OA over 36 months (compared to a neutral insole) [33], this study has only been reported in an abstract form. Further longitudinal research using magnetic resonance imaging of cartilage changes is required to evaluate the effects of lateral wedges on disease course.

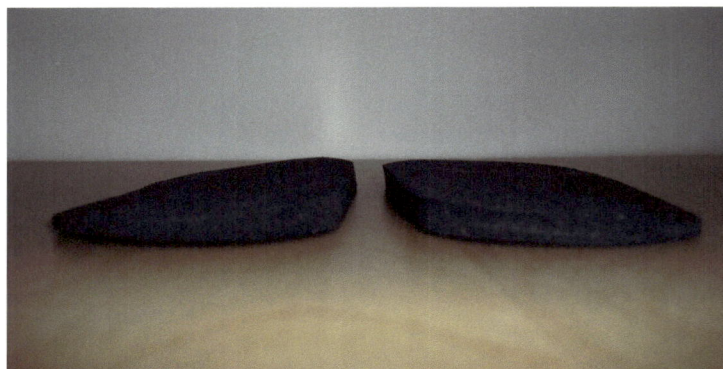

Figure 2: A typical pair of medial wedged insoles. Note these insoles are wedged along the full length of the foot and are inclined approximately 5°.

2.4. Medial Wedged Insoles for Lateral Tibiofemoral Osteoarthritis

In contrast to lateral wedged insoles, there is very little research evaluating medial wedged insoles (Fig. **2**) for lateral compartment knee OA. Interest in medial wedged insoles arose when a case series involving 10 patients with lateral knee OA reported that medial wedges reduced lateral thrust and pain in walking [21]. Confirming these early findings, a more recent study in 10 healthy people showed that medial wedges attached to the sole of the shoe alone or combined with ankle orthoses altered frontal knee loading favourably for the lateral knee compartment [34]. Unfortunately, little is known about the effects of medial wedged insoles on knee OA symptoms however the limited evidence available is favourable. In the only randomised controlled trial conducted (Table **1**), improved pain and function, together with improved femorotibial angle, was observed with a rearfoot medial wedge worn with an ankle support for eight weeks (compared to a neutral insole) in women with valgus lateral compartment OA [35]. This supports the use of medial wedges for predominant lateral compartment OA but further research into medial wedges is needed to validate these findings and to identify which patient subgroups will most benefit from treatment. There is no data available regarding the effect of medial wedges on structural disease progression over time.

2.5. Biomechanical Effects of Medial Arch Supports

Although medial arch supports are widely available (Fig. **3**), and are probably the most commonly used type of insole in people with knee OA, there is no research evaluating their effects in people with this condition. Evidence from healthy people suggests that medial arch supports could in fact be detrimental in medial tibiofemoral OA as they may shift the centre of pressure medially, thereby increasing the knee adduction moment. A recent study showed that flexible medial arch supports resulted in a 6% increase in the second peak knee adduction moment during walking in young healthy people [36]. Interestingly, medial arch supports used in combination with lateral wedged insoles may enhance effects of the wedge on the knee adduction moment [37]. It is unclear why this is the case, but may be related to effects of the combined insole on step width and/or foot progression angle. Until the effects of medial arch supports are evaluated in people with medial OA, they should be used cautiously in this patient population.

3. EFFECT OF FOOTWEAR ON KNEE LOADING AND OA SYMPTOMS

Clinical guidelines recommend that patients with knee OA wear appropriate footwear [18]. However, due to limited research, this recommendation is based solely on expert opinion and there is little data available to guide patients and clinicians regarding optimal footwear choices. With the exception of research commenced by Kerrigan and colleagues 10 years ago [38-41], most research into the potential role of shoes for knee OA has been conducted only in the past few years. A proportion of this work is available only in abstract form. Other limitations of the current body of evidence include the use of younger healthy individuals without OA, primarily biomechanical evaluations addressing effects of shoes on loading rather than symptoms and a dearth of randomized controlled trials (Table **2**).

3.1. Effect of Shoes on Knee Joint Loading Compared to Bare Feet

Two studies evaluating patients with knee OA have shown that wearing shoes significantly increases medial knee load compared to walking in barefeet. The most recent study examined the everyday shoes of 40 people with medial compartment OA [42]. Compared to walking barefooted, wearing shoes resulted in a 7.4% increase in the knee adduction moment. These findings were in agreement with those of an earlier study [43]. Changes in joint loading when wearing shoes do not seem to be caused by changes in gait pattern because of shoes [43]. This would suggest that the design of everyday off-the-shelf shoes may potentially predispose knee OA patients to excessive joint loading. This hypothesis is supported by data demonstrating that the effect of shoes on knee loads is not systematic. For example, although most participants in the study by Kemp *et al.* [42] demonstrated an increased knee adduction moment with shoes, considerable individual variation was observed, with 15% of individuals showing reduced knee loading with shoes and some showing increased loading by 20-30% (compared to barefoot), far in excess of the average 7.4% increase demonstrated by the entire cohort. It therefore seems likely that individual shoe characteristics may mediate effects of footwear on knee loading. Based on research showing that a one-unit increase in the adduction moment increases the risk of OA progression 6.5 times [44], the more conservative findings of Kemp *et al.* [42] suggest that wearing shoes may increase the risk of knee OA progression by a factor of 2.8 on average.

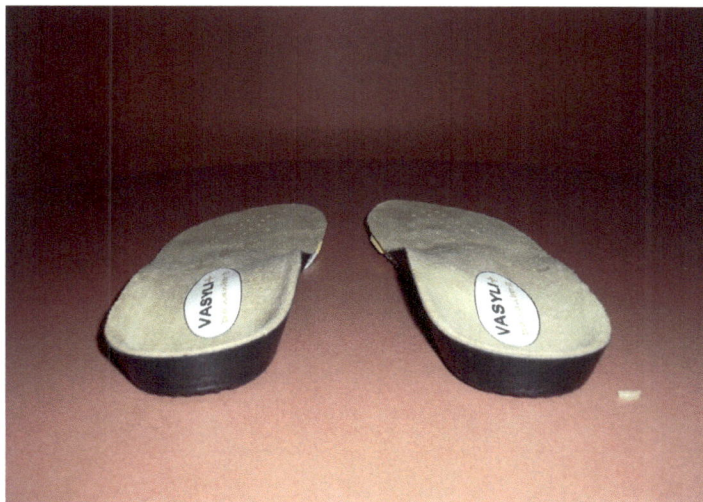

Figure 3: An example of commercially available medial arch support insoles.

3.2. Off-the-Shelf Shoes and Their Effects on Knee Load

Current research suggests that some types of off-the-shelf shoes may increase knee loads more than others. Heel height appears to be an important factor in explaining the increased knee loads observed with footwear. Studies in healthy women without knee OA have shown that walking in high-heeled shoes (approximately 2.5-2.8 inch) resulted in greater loads across the medial knee compartment and the patellofemoral joint compared to barefoot [41], irrespective of heel width [40].

Although a flat-heeled comparison shoe was not included in these initial studies, subsequent research demonstrated that moderate-heeled (approximately 1.5 inch) shoes resulted 9-14% increases in late stance varus knee torque (adduction moment) in younger and older healthy women compared to flat-heeled control shoes [38]. In contrast, men's dress shoes and sneakers, with an average heel height of 0.5 inch, did not significantly influence joint torques (other than that explained by changes in walking speed) compared to barefoot walking [39]. These findings suggest that shoes with a heel of >1.5 inch may detrimentally influence medial knee load and should be avoided or worn minimally by patients with medial knee OA. These findings concur with the randomized controlled trial discussed earlier that evaluated the effects of concomitant heeled footwear on outcome with lateral wedged insoles [15] (Table **2**), and found greater improvements in symptoms when insoles were worn in combination with barefeet or flat-heeled shoes. The long-term effects of wearing high-heeled shoes on disease incidence and progression remain unknown, as is their effect on knee symptoms.

Table 1: Summary of randomised controlled trials (RCTs) evaluating the symptomatic efficacy of insoles for knee osteoarthritis (OA).

References	Design	Population	Intervention	Follow-up	Outcomes measured	Results
Toda *et al.* (2001) [27]	Quasi-RCT	Female adults ≥45 years with ACR diagnosed knee OA (n=90)	1) Lateral urethane heel wedges (6.35mm elevation) strapped to an ankle sprain supporter + daily oral NSAID 2) Lateral rubber heel wedge (6.35 mm elevation) inserted into own shoes + daily oral NSAID	8 weeks	Lequesne index Knee pain (VAS) TC, TF & TT angles on xray	Improvements in Lequesne index were similar in each group, but strapped insoles reduced pain more than inserted insoles. Strapped insoles produced significant changes in all angles while inserted insole only changed TC angle.
Toda & Segal (2002) [16]	Quasi-RCT	Female adults with ACR diagnosed knee OA (n=88)	1) Lateral urethane heel wedge (6.35mm elevation) fixed to an ankle strap + daily oral NSAID 2) Sock-type ankle supporter with lateral rubber heel wedge insert (6.35 mm elevation) + daily oral NSAID	8 weeks	Lequesne index TF angle on xray	Strapped insole improved symptoms (pain, distance walked and aggregate severity score) and decreased TF angle while sock insole only improved aggregate severity score.
Toda & Tsukimura (2004) [28] Toda & Tsukimura (2006) [29]	Quasi-RCT	Female adults with ACR diagnosed medial knee OA and varus deformity (n=66)	1) Lateral urethane heel wedges (12mm elevation/11.2° tilt) fixed to an ankle sprain supporter + daily oral NSAID 2) Lateral rubber heel wedge (6.35 mm elevation/5° tilt) inserted into own shoes + daily oral NSAID	6 months 2 years	Lequesne index Knee pain (VAS) TF angle on xray Radiographic progression on xray	Decreased TF angle and improved knee pain and Lequesne scores at 6 months & 2 years with the strapped insole, whereas no such changes were seen with the inserted insole. No differences in radiographic progression were detected across groups.

Maillefert *et al.* (2001) [23] Pham *et al.* (2004) [24]	RCT	Adults >18 years with xray & symptomatic medial TF OA (n=156)	1) Bilateral individually modelled laterally wedged (rear foot) insoles 2) Bilateral neutrally wedged insoles	1 month 3 months 6 months 2 years	Patient's overall assessment of disease activity WOMAC Analgesic & NSAID use Medial JSW Compliance	No difference between groups regarding symptoms or JSW. Reduced NSAID intake and better compliance in favour of a beneficial effect of lateral wedges.
Baker *et al.* (2007) [53]	Randomised crossover trial	Adults >50 years with knee pain & medial TF narrowing on xray (n=90)	1) Non-custom 5° lateral-wedge insole on the side with knee OA 2) Flat neutral insole on the side with knee OA	3 weeks 6 weeks	WOMAC Overall knee pain (VAS) Physical performance measures Analgesic & NSAID use	No differences between groups on any outcome.
Rodrigues *et al.* (2008) [35]	RCT	Women with lateral compartment xray changes of OA, knee pain and bilateral valgus deformity ≥8° (n=30)	1) Medial wedge rearfoot insole (8mm high) and elastic ankle support worn in new shoes 2) Neutral insole and elastic ankle support worn in new shoes	8 weeks	Knee pain (VAS) Lequesne index WOMAC	The medial wedge resulted in greater improvements in knee pain, WOMAC and Lequesne scores compared to the neutral insole.
Toda & Tsukimura (2008) [15]	RCT	Adults with ACR diagnosed medial knee OA and varus deformity (n=227)	1) Neutral (placebo) insole inserted into own regular shoes 2) Lateral rubber heel wedge (6.35 mm elevation/5° tilt) inserted into own shoes 3) Sock-type ankle supporter with the lateral rubber heel wedge sewn into it and worn with socks only or flat shoes without any heel 4) Lateral urethane heel wedges (12mm elevation/11.2° tilt) fixed to an ankle sprain supporter and used with socks or flat shoes 5) Lateral urethane heel wedges (12mm elevation/11.2° tilt) fixed to an ankle sprain supporter and used with own shoes	3 months	Lequesne index Knee pain (VAS)	Improvements in Lequesne index and knee pain over time were noted only with the strapped insoles and own shoes, the strapped insoles with socks/flat shoes and the inserted insoles with socks/flat shoes (Lequesne index only).
Barrios *et al.* (2009) [26]	RCT	Adults aged 40-75 years with xray & symptomatic medial TF OA (n=66)	1) Standardised walking shoe with individually-prescribed (5-15°) full-length lateral wedging applied to a neutral contoured foot orthosis on the most symptomatic side with knee OA 2) Standardised walking shoe with non-custom pair of neutral contoured foot orthoses	1 month 1 year	WOMAC Physical performance measures Pain during physical performance tasks (VAS)	Both groups demonstrated similar improvements in outcomes, however only the lateral wedge group showed early improvements in walking test pain.

ACR=American College of Rheumatology; TF=tibiofemoral; WOMAC= Western Ontario and McMaster Universities Index; NSAID=non-steroidal anti-inflammatory drugs; JSW=joint space width; TC=talocalcaneal; TT=talar tilt; VAS=visual analogue scale.

Only one other study has directly compared off-the-shelf shoe types. Four common shoe types (clogs, stability athletic shoes, flexible walking shoes and flip-flops) were compared to barefoot walking in a small cohort with knee OA [45]. Both clogs and stability athletic shoes significantly increased the knee adduction moment compared to barefoot, whilst the flexible walking shoes and flip-flops had no effect. Thus, it appears that flexible footwear better approximates barefoot walking and may minimize knee loading. Further research is required to determine which off-the-shelf shoe types are optimal for knee OA and to evaluate their long-term effects on symptoms and disease progression.

3.3. Footwear Modifications Relevant to Knee OA

As there is no commercially available shoe proven to reduce medial knee compartment load, increasing research is focused on developing and evaluating shoes that are designed specifically to reduce the knee adduction moment. One such shoe is the "mobility" shoe. The mobility shoe is a flexible light-weight shoe designed to mimic barefoot walking *via* specialized grooves in the sole placed at major foot flexion points [46, 47]. Data from participants with knee OA show that the knee adduction moment recorded with the mobility shoe approximates that of barefoot walking. It can significantly reduce the adduction moment by 12% compared to a control shoe and by 8% compared to conventional self-selected walking shoes. It remains to be seen whether the immediate reductions in knee load evident with the mobility shoe can be maintained with prolonged use over the longer-term and whether biomechanical benefits translate into improvements in symptoms.

Another shoe with relevance to knee OA is the "unstable" shoe, manufactured by Masai Barefoot Technology®. Unstable shoes have been designed to strengthen lower extremity muscles that contribute to static and dynamic stability [48, 49]. The shoe has a multilayered sole that changes flat hard surfaces into uneven ground, demanding increased muscle activity from the lower limb in order to maintain stability. A small study in young healthy people showed that unstable shoes produced kinematic, kinetic and electromyographic changes deemed to be advantageous [49]. A 12-week randomized controlled trial conducted in 123 people with knee OA compared unstable shoes to off-the-shelf walking shoes [48] (Table 2). Both groups demonstrated reductions in knee pain with generally no differences between the two shoe types tested. While there were trends towards improved balance performance in the group wearing unstable shoes, differences were not significant between groups. Furthermore, no differences between groups regarding joint motion or strength were observed. At this stage, a specially designed unstable shoe appears to offer little clinical benefit to patients with knee OA.

Based on the promising results of inserted lateral wedged insoles, some studies have evaluated the effects of shoes modified to incorporate a laterally angled sole. Such a shoe has advantages as it may overcome the difficulties experienced by patients when inserting the wedged insole into their usual shoes, such as foot blistering and discomfort, because of the reduced space inside the shoe once the insole is inserted.

In young healthy adults, Fisher *et al.* [50] demonstrated that shoes with either a 4° or 8° valgus shoe sole angle significantly reduced the knee adduction moment compared to a control shoe with no angulation. In contrast, another study that attached a 14° wedge to the shoe did not reduce the varus knee moment unless combined with a rigid ankle stabilizing orthosis [34]. It is not clear why results of these studies differ but differences in the type of shoe used or the length of the sole wedging may be responsible. Modifications to shoe sole stiffness have also been tested for their potential application to knee OA. A variable-stiffness mid-sole that is more dense (rigid) laterally than medially can significantly reduce the adduction moment in healthy young adults compared to control shoes of uniform sole stiffness [50]. Data from older individuals with medial knee OA shows similar results. Erhart *et al.* [51] tested a variable-stiffness shoe in 79 people with medial OA and found average reductions in the knee adduction moment ranging from 2.2% to 6.2%, depending on walking speed and compared to a constant-stiffness control shoe. Importantly, reductions in the knee adduction moment did not occur at the expense of overloading other lower joints. Further data from a randomized controlled trial showed improvements in pain and function at 6 months with variable-stiffness shoes compared to control shoes [52]. Thus it seems that variable-stiffness shoes offer great potential for medial knee OA and should be subjected to further larger clinical trials that include measures of structural disease progression.

CONCLUDING REMARKS

There is considerable evidence that excessive joint loading significantly increases the risk of disease progression in people with knee OA. Increasing research demonstrates that such excessive knee loading may be amenable to change in most individuals with knee OA *via* the use of insoles and/or footwear. Accordingly, insoles and footwear offer great potential as simple, inexpensive treatment strategies for knee OA. Current research suggests that lateral wedged insoles are beneficial in reducing knee load in people with medial tibiofemoral OA, whilst medial wedged insoles are more suitable for those with lateral compartment disease. However, biomechanical benefits of lateral wedged insoles do not seem to incur any symptomatic benefit. Further research is needed to evaluate the efficacy of wedged insoles in relieving OA-associated symptoms and whether biomechanical benefits translate into a reduced risk of disease progression.

Table 2: Summary of randomised controlled trials (RCTs) evaluating the symptomatic efficacy of footwear for knee osteoarthritis (OA).

References	Design	Population	Intervention	Follow-up	Outcomes measured	Results
Nigg *et al.* (2006) [48]	RCT	Adults >40 years with symptomatic and xray changes of OA (n=123)	1) Masai Barefoot Technology® shoes ('unstable' shoe) 2) Walking shoes	3 weeks 6 weeks 9 weeks 12 weeks	WOMAC Balance Active range of motion Ankle torque	Both groups exhibited similar reductions in pain at all times, except between 3 and 6 weeks where the unstable shoe resulted in greater pain reduction. No other between group differences were detected for any other measure.
Toda & Tsukimura (2008) [15]	RCT	Adults with ACR diagnosed medial knee OA and varus deformity (n=227)	1) Neutral (placebo) insole inserted into own regular shoes 2) Lateral rubber heel wedge (6.35 mm elevation/5° tilt) inserted into own shoes 3) Sock-type ankle supporter with the lateral rubber heel wedge sewn into it and worn with socks only or flat shoes without any heel 4) Lateral urethane heel wedges (12mm elevation/11.2° tilt) fixed to an ankle sprain supporter and used with socks or flat shoes 5) Lateral urethane heel wedges (12mm elevation/11.2° tilt) fixed to an ankle sprain supporter and used with own shoes	3 months	Lequesne index Knee pain (VAS)	Improvements in Lequesne index and knee pain over time were noted only with the strapped insoles and own shoes, the strapped insoles with socks/flat shoes and the inserted insoles with socks/flat shoes (Lequesne index only).
Erhart *et al.* (2010) [52]	RCT	Medial compartment knee OA (n=60)	1) Variable stiffness sole shoe 2) Constant stiffness sole shoe	6 months	WOMAC Knee adduction moment	There was no difference between groups in magnitude of the reduction in total WOMAC or WOMAC pain scores. The proportion of patients achieving a clinically important improvement in pain was greater in the intervention group than in the control group. The variable-stiffness shoes reduced the peak knee adduction moment at 6 months. The adduction moment reduction significantly improved from the baseline reduction.

Research is also required to determine which patient subgroups are most likely to respond to treatment. Given that shoe heel height influences medial compartment knee load, patients with knee OA should be encouraged to wear flat-heeled shoes as much as possible, in preference to those with a heel >1.5 inches in height. It appears that flexible shoes promoting mobility may be preferable to supportive shoes promoting stability [54]. Further research into the effects of different shoe types on knee pain and disease progression are needed to help guide clinical decision making.

ACKNOWLEDGEMENTS

The authors have received funding from ASICS Oceania Pty Ltd to develop and evaluate a modified shoe for Osteoarthritis.

REFERENCES

[1] Sasaki T, Yasuda K. Clinical evaluation of the treatment of osteoarthritic knees using a newly designed wedged insole. Clin Orthop 1987; 221:181-7.

[2] Yasuda K, Sasaki T. The mechanics of treatment of the osteoarthritic knee with a wedged insole. Clin Orthop 1987; 215:162-72.

[3] Ledingham J, Regan M, Jones A, Doherty M. Radiographic patterns and associations of osteoarthritis of the knee in patients referred to hospital. Ann Rheum Dis 1993; 52: 520-6.

[4] Butler R, Marchesi S, Royer T, Davis I. The effect of a subject-specific amount of lateral wedge on knee mechanics in patients with medial knee osteoarthritis. J Orthop Res 2007; 25:1121-7.

[5] Hinman R, Bowles K, Payne C, Bennell K. Effect of length on laterally wedged insoles in knee osteoarthritis. Arthritis Rheum (Arthritis Care Res) 2008; 59: 144-7.

[6] Hinman R, Payne C, Metcalf B, Wrigley T, Bennell K. Lateral wedges in knee osteoarthritis: what are their immediate clinical and biomechanical effects and can these predict a three-month clinical outcome? Arthritis Rheum (Arthritis Care Res) 2008; 59: 408-15.

[7] Kakihana W, Akai M, Nakazawa K, Takashima T, Naito K, Torii S. Effects of laterally wedged insoles on knee and subtalar joint moments. Arch Phys Med Rehabil 2005; 86: 1465-71.

[8] Kerrigan D, Lelas J, Goggins J, Merriman G, Kaplan R, Felson D. Effectiveness of a lateral-wedge insole on knee varus torque in patients with knee osteoarthritis. Arch Phys Med Rehabil 2002;83:889-93.

[9] Kuroyanagi Y, Nagura T, Matsumoto H, *et al.* The lateral wedged insole with subtalar strapping significantly reduces dynamic knee load in the medial compartment- gait analysis on patients with medial knee osteoarthritis. Osteoarthritis Cartilage 2007; 15: 932-6.

[10] Shimada S, Kobayashi S, Wada M, *et al.* Effects of disease severity on response to lateral wedged shoe insole for medial compartment knee osteoarthritis. Arch Phys Med Rehabil 2006; 87: 1436-41.

[11] Shelburne K, Torry M, Steadman J, Pandy MG. Effects of foot orthoses and valgus bracing on the knee adduction moment and medial joint load during gait. Clinical Biomechanics 2008; 23: 814-21.

[12] Thorp L, Wimmer M, Sumner D, Lidtke R, Block J. Custom shoe inserts induce beneficial long-term gait adaptations in medial knee osteoarthritis. Arthritis Rheum 2007; 56: S120.

[13] Kakihana W, Akai M, Nakazawa K, Naito K, Torii S. Inconsistent knee varus moment reduction caused by a lateral wedge in knee osteoarthritis. Am J Phys Med Rehabil 2007; 86: 446-54.

[14] Lidtke R, Muehleman C, Foucher K, Wimmer M, Block J. Motion at rearfoot determines if valgus wedged orthosis reduces knee adduction moments in medial knee osteoarthritis. Arthritis Rheumatism 2006; 54: S670.

[15] Toda Y, Tsukimura N. Influence of concomitant heeled footwear when wearing a lateral wedged insole for medial compartment osteoarthritis of the knee. Osteoarthritis Cartilage 2008; 16: 244-53.

[16] Toda Y, Segal N. Usefulness of an insole with subtalar strapping for analgesia in patients with medial compartment osteoarthritis of the knee. Arthritis Care Res 2002; 47: 468-73.

[17] Butler R, Barrios J, Royer T, Davis I. Effect of laterally wedged foot orthoses on rearfoot and hip mechanics in patients with medial knee osteoarthritis. Prosthet Orthot Int 2009; 33:107-16.

[18] Zhang W, Moskowitz R, Nuki G, *et al.* OARSI recommendations for the management of hip and knee osteoarthritis. Part II: OARSI evidence-based, expert consensus guidelines. Osteoarthritis Cartilage 2008;16:137-62.

[19] Fang M, Taylor C, Nouvong A, Masih S, Kao K, Perell K. Effects of footwear on medial compartment knee osteoarthritis. J Rehabil Res Devel 2006; 43: 427-34.

[20] Keating E, Faris P, Ritter M, Kane J. Use of lateral heel and sole wedges in the treatment of medial osteoarthritis of the knee. Orthop Rev 1993; 22: 921-4.

[21] Ogata K, Yasunaga M, Nomiyama H. The effect of wedged insoles on the thrust of osteoarthritic knees. Int Orthop 1997; 21: 308-12.

[22] Tohyama H, Yasuda K, Kaneda K. Treatment of osteoarthritis of the knee with heel wedges. Int Orthop 1991;15:31-3.

[23] Maillefert J, Hudry C, Baron G, *et al.* Laterally elevated wedged insoles in the treatment of medial knee osteoarthritis: a prospective randomised controlled study. Osteoarthritis Cartilage 2001; 9: 738-45.

[24] Pham T, Maillefert J, Hudry C, *et al.* Laterally elevated wedged insoles in the treatment of medial knee osteoarthritis. A two year prospective randomized controlled study. Osteoarthritis Cartilage 2003; 12: 46-55.

[25] Baker K, Goggins J, Xie H, *et al.* A randomized crossover trial of a wedged insole for treatment of knee osteoarthritis. Arthritis Rheum 2007; 56: 1198-203.

[26] Barrios J, Crenshaw J, Royer T, Davis I. Walking shoes and laterally wedged orthoses in the clinical management of medial tibiofemoral osteoarthritis: a one-year prospective controlled trial. Knee 2009; 16: 136-42.

[27] Toda Y, Segal N, Kato A, Yamamoto S, Irie M. Effect of a novel insole on the subtalar joint of patients with medial compartment osteoarthritis of the knee. J Rheumatol 2001; 28: 2705-10.

[28] Toda Y, Tsukimura N. A six-month followup of a randomized trial comparing the efficacy of a lateral-wedge insole with subtalar strapping and an in-shoe lateral-wedge insole in patients with varus deformity osteoarthritis of the knee. Arthritis Rheum 2004; 50: 3129-36.

[29] Toda Y, Tsukimura N. A 2-year follow-up of a study to compare the efficacy of lateral wedged insoles with subtalar strapping and in-shoe lateral wedged insoles in patients with varus deformity osteoarthritis of the knee. Osteoarthritis Cartilage 2006; 14: 231-7.

[30] Brouwer R, Jakma T, Verhagen A, Verhaar J, Bierma-Zeinstra S. Braces and orthoses for treating osteoarthritis of the knee. Cochrane Libr 2005; 1.

[31] Toda Y, Segal N, Kato A, Yamamoto S, Irie M. Correlation between body composition and efficacy of lateral wedged insoles for medial compartment osteoarthritis of the knee. J Rheumatol 2002; 29: 541-5.

[32] Toda Y, Tsukimura N, Segal N. An optimal duration of daily wear for an insole with subtalar strapping in patients with varus deformity osteoarthritis of the knee. Osteoarthritis Cartilage 2005; 13: 353-60.

[33] Goker B, Demirag M, Block J. Lateral wedge orthotics delay progression of joint space narrowing in patients with medial knee osteoarthritis. Arthritis Rheum 2008; 58: S241.

[34] Schmalz T, Blumentritt S, Drewitz H, Freslier M. The influence of sole wedges on frontal plane kinetics, in isolation and in combination with representative rigid and semi-rigid ankle-foot-orthoses. Clin Biomech 2006; 21: 631-9.

[35] Rodrigues P, Ferreira A, Pereira R, Bonfa E, Borba E, Fuller R. Effectiveness of medial-wedge insole treatment for valgus knee osteoarthritis. Arthritis Rheum (Arthritis Care Res) 2008; 59: 603-8.

[36] Franz J, Dicharry J, Riley P, Jackson K, Wilder R, Kerrigan D. The influence of arch supports on knee torques relevant to knee osteoarthritis. Med Sci Sports Exer 2008; 40: 913-7.

[37] Nakajima K, Kakihana W, Nakagawa T, *et al.* Addition of an arch support improves the biomechanical effect of a laterally wedged insole. Gait Posture 2009; 29: 208-13.

[38] Kerrigan D, Johansson J, Bryant M, Boxer J, Della Croce U, Riley P. Moderate-heeled shoes and knee joint torques relevant to the development and progression of knee osteoarthritis. Arch Phys Med Rehabil 2005; 86: 871-5.

[39] Kerrigan D, Karvosky M, Lelas J, Riley P. Men's shoes and knee joint torques relevant to the development and progression of knee osteoarthritis. J Rheumatol 2003; 30: 529-33.

[40] Kerrigan D, Lelas J, Karvosky M. Women's shoes and knee osteoarthritis. Lancet 2001; 357: 1097-8.

[41] Kerrigan DC, Todd MK, Riley PO. Knee osteoarthritis and high-heeled shoes. Lancet 1998; 351: 1399-401.

[42] Kemp G, Crossley K, Wrigley T, Metcalf B, Hinman R. Reducing joint loading in medial knee osteoarthritis: shoes and canes. Arthritis Care Res 2008; 59: 609-14.

[43] Shakoor N, Block J. Walking barefoot decreases loading on the lower extremity joints in knee osteoarthritis. Arthritis Rheum 2006; 54: 2923-7.

[44] Miyazaki T, Wada M, Kawahara H, Sato M, Baba H, Shimada S. Dynamic load at baseline can predict radiographic disease progression in medial compartment knee osteoarthritis. Ann Rheum Dis 2002; 61: 617-22.

[45] Shakoor N, Sengupta M, Foucher KC *et al.* Effects of common footwear on joint loading in osteoarthritis of the knee. Arthritis Care Res 2010; 62: 917-23.

[46]   Shakoor N, Lidtke R, Sengupta M, Trombley R, Block J. "Mobility" footwear reduces dynamic loads in subjects with osteoarthritis of the knee. Osteoarthritis Cartilage 2007; 15: C219.

[47]   Shakoor N, Lidtke RH, Sengupta M, Fogg LF, Block JA. Effects of specialized footwear on joint loads in osteoarthritis of the knee. Arthritis Rheum 2008; 59: 1214-20.

[48]   Nigg B, Emery C, Hiemstra L. Unstable shoe construction and reduction of pain in osteoarthritis patients. Med Sci Sports Exerc 2006; 38: 1701-8.

[49].   Nigg B, Hintzen S, Ferber R. Effect of an unstable shoe construction on lower extremity gait characterstics. Clin Biomech 2006; 21: 82-8.

[50]   Fisher D, Dyrby C, Mundermann A, Morag E, Andriacchi T. In healthy subjects without knee osteoarthritis, the peak knee adduction moment influences the acute effect of shoe interventions designed to reduce medial compartment knee load. J Orthop Res 2007; 25: 540-6.

[51]   Erhart J, Mundermann A, Elspas B, Giori N, Andriacchi T. A variable-stiffness shoe lowers the knee adduction moment in subjects with symptoms of medial compartment knee osteoarthritis. J Biomech 2008; 41: 2720-5.

[52]   Erhart J, Mundermann A, Elspas B *et al*. Changes in knee adduction moment, pain, and functionality with a variable-stiffness walking shoe after 6 months. J Orthop Res 2010; 28: 873-9.

[53]   Baker K, Goggins J, Xie, *et al*. A randomized cross-over trial of a wedged insole for treatment of knee osteoarthritis. Arthritis Rheum 2007; 56: 1198-1203.

[54]   Hinman RS, Bennell KL. Adavances in insoles and shoes for knee OA. Curr Opin Rheumatol 2009; 21(2):164-70.

CHAPTER 10

Nutraceuticals: From Research to Legal and Regulatory Affairs

A. Mobasheri[1*], K. Asplin[1], A. Clutterbuck[1] and M. Shakibaei[2]

[1]*Musculoskeletal Research Group, School of Veterinary Medicine and Science, Faculty of Medicine and Health Sciences, University of Nottingham, Sutton Bonington Campus, Sutton Bonington, LE12 5RD, United Kingdom and* [2]*Musculoskeletal Research Group, Institute of Anatomy, Ludwig-Maximilians-University Munich, D-80336 Munich, Germany*

Abstract: In this chapter we define the term "nutraceutical" and its relevance to arthritic diseases, and summarize recent research on nutraceuticals for joint disorders, particularly osteoarthritis (OA). The nutraceutical industry is not regulated. Consequently there are concerns about the purity, labeling and advertising of nutraceuticals. Manufacturers of nutraceuticals have a duty to communicate the benefits of their products with supporting scientific and clinical evidence. Nutraceutical products should be clearly labelled and advertising campaigns should be truthful and well balanced. The public and the scientific community require greater transparency and uniformity of commercially produced nutraceuticals. Consumers need to be able to make an informed choice about nutraceuticals based on evidence. We advocate greater regulation and regular independent testing of these products in order to ensure uniformity and greater reliability. The intended audience for this article include clinicians, basic researchers, producers of nutraceuticals and functional foods and advertising and marketing companies worldwide, particularly multi-national companies requiring information on issues relating to nutraceutical regulation.

Keywords: Osteoarthritis (OA), nutraceutical, regulation, purity, labeling, advertising.

1. INTRODUCTION

"Nutraceutical" is a term originally coined by Stephen L. DeFelice in 1989 when he combined the words "nutrition" and "pharmaceutical". An attempt was made by Ekta K. Kalra in 2003 to redefine the terms "nutraceutical" and "functional food" [1]. But the revised definitions were introduced to distinguish between functional foods, nutraceuticals, and dietary supplements the basic definition has not changed since its introduction. When a functional food aids in the prevention and/or treatment of a disease or disorder it is called a nutraceutical [1]. Nutraceuticals are nutritional products that claim to provide medicinal benefits over and above their basic nutritional value. In essence a nutraceutical is "any food or food ingredient which is considered to have a beneficial effect on health".

"The Nutraceutical Revolution" (see footnotes[1] and[2]) as defined by DeFelice is a powerful new international market, which is predicted to grow substantially over the next few decades, approaching the size of the pharmaceutical market. The term "nutraceutical" has been adopted by the food marketing industry to describe any food, food derived product, dietary supplement, medical food or functional food that may have a functional or physiological effect that may be beneficial to health or prevent and treat illness or disease. Therefore the description "nutraceutical" is very broadly used and can refer to anything from a vitamin supplement pill to an energy enhancing drink and more recently to foods which are claimed to have physiological effects. Although nutraceuticals are classed as food products, use of the term nutraceutical and the claims attributed to the properties of the product have lead to some confusion as to whether nutraceuticals should be classed as medicinal products. The current consensus is that nutraceuticals

***Address correspondence to A. Mobasheri:** Division of Veterinary Medicine, School of Veterinary Medicine and Science, Faculty of Medicine and Health Sciences, University of Nottingham, Sutton Bonington Campus, Sutton Bonington, Leicestershire, LE12 5RD, United Kingdom; Tel.: +44 115 951 6449; Fax: +44 115 951 6440; E-mail address: ali.mobasheri@nottingham.ac.uk
[1] http://www.fimdefelice.org/archives/arc.fueling.html
[1] http://www.fimdefelice.org/clippings/clip.future.html

Yves Henrotin, Kim Bennell and Francois Rannou (Eds)

are not covered by the provision of s130(2) Medicines Act 1968 which states that a medicinal product is a substance or ingredient used in the preparation of a substance which is administered for a medicinal purpose where a medicinal purpose is defined as the following:

- treating, preventing or diagnosing disease;

- contraception; or

- inducing anaesthesia.

2. THE RISE OF NUTRACEUTICALS AND ALTERNATIVE MEDICINES

The advent of food-derived nutraceuticals has revolutionized the concept of 'self-prescribed' and 'personalized' medicine for humans [2, 3]. Many patients with arthritis freely purchase and consume well-known nutraceuticals including glucosamine sulfate, chondroitin sulfate, vitamin C and essential oils, in addition to medically prescribed Non-Steroidal Anti-Inflammatory Drugs (NSAIDs). Companion animals are also benefiting from advances in nutraceutical research. In recent years there has been a proliferation of research into plant extracts with potential anti-inflammatory properties [4, 5]. The most important factor that drives the interest in nutraceuticals, functional foods and botanical extracts is the realization that inflammation plays a central role in the development of many chronic diseases in humans and animals. Consequently researchers working on many diverse diseases with a core inflammatory component are embracing the concept of nutraceuticals and alternative medicines. However, this is not a novel concept; for example the use of plant extracts to alleviate inflammatory disease is widespread in Indian, Chinese and Korean traditional medicine. A number of plant extracts have been reported to protect against mutagenesis and carcinogenesis [6-12]. Plant-extracts and plant-derived agents have also been shown to possess strong anti-inflammatory and anti-arthritic properties [4, 5, 13-23]. Therefore, practices that were common centuries ago are being revisited today [24]. Since OA and related osteoarticular conditions of synovial joints are characterized by inflammation, a better understanding of the nutritional biochemistry of various different alternative medicines and nutraceuticals and their biological actions in joint tissues may facilitate the development of clinically safe, orally administered therapeutic agents for preventing and treating joint diseases.

The growing interest in alternative medicines and nutraceuticals may reflect a general and increasing disenchantment with traditional medicine. This could be due to a number of factors: conventional treatment may not be working as well as patients would like; patients want greater relief of symptoms and/or disability; they have issues with side-effects of pharmaceutical treatment; they wish to reduce some of the stress that comes from living with a chronic illness and want to cope better; they believe that complementary and alternative therapies are safer and 'natural'; and they are influenced by the widespread advertising and attractive claims that are made for many natural products. Another reason why people use complementary and alternative medicine could be the corruption and gradual degradation of 'managed care' and the classic patient-physician relationship. When in comes to chronic and difficult to cure diseases, such as cancer, much of it may be frustration at the inability of modern scientific medicine to overcome disease, and an increase in patient outspokenness and access to medical information. A few managed care plans cover some forms of alternative medicine in the hope that patients will select them as less expensive treatment options.

Within the realm of alternative medicine, nutraceuticals represent one of the boldest challenges to various government and state regulations. In 1992 the National Institutes of Health (NIH) established an Office of Alternative Medicine. The United States Congress subsequently elevated this to a Center for Complementary and Alternative Medicine with a multi-million dollar annual budget. Historically, the U S Food and Drug Administration (FDA) took the view that a product that made health claims was a drug. Consequently in the 1970s vitamins and minerals were exempted from regulation as drugs as long as they did not make health claims. In the early 1980s, studies demonstrated that certain food ingredients, such as fibre, provided specific benefits to health. Food manufacturers wanted to proclaim these benefits to consumers without having to obtain drug approval. The FDA wrestled with this problem until the US

Congress passed the Nutrition Labeling and Education Act of 1990. This law authorized the FDA to issue regulations permitting certain health claims for foods, which led the agency to allow claims associating low levels of calcium with osteoporosis, dietary fats with cancer and cholesterol with heart disease. After passage of the FDA Modernization Act of 1997, a food could make a health claim without FDA regulatory authority so long as the claim was based on an authoritative statement by a governmental or quasi-governmental scientific body (such as the NIH or the National Academy of Science [NAS]) and the agency was given advanced notice of the manufacturer's intent. However, this leeway did not apply to dietary supplements and so it resulted in much confusion. Clearly, this is an area that is constantly changing and evolving but it still requires regulation and monitoring. It is beyond the scope of this chapter to provide a global history of the development and evolution of alternative medicines and nutraceuticals. The aim of this chapter is to summarize the current state of the field in the context of OA and inflammatory joint diseases and highlight some of the problems with the regulation of nutraceuticals.

3. OSTEOARTHRITIS (OA)

According to the World Health Organization (WHO) musculoskeletal conditions are leading causes of morbidity and disability, giving rise to enormous healthcare expenditures and loss of work throughout the world (source: http://www.arthritis.org/)[3, 4]. OA is one of the most prevalent and chronic diseases affecting the elderly [25]. Its most prominent feature is the progressive destruction of articular cartilage [26]. The current consensus is that OA is a disease involving not only articular cartilage but also the synovial membrane, subchondral bone and peri-articular soft tissues [27]. OA may occur following traumatic injury to the joint, subsequent to an infection of the joint or simply as a result of aging and the mechanical stresses associated with daily life.

The symptoms and signs characteristic of OA in the most frequently affected joints are heat, swelling, pain, stiffness and limited mobility. Other sequelae include osteophyte formation and joint mal-alignment. These manifestations are highly variable, depending on joint location and disease severity.

It is now generally accepted that OA must be viewed not only as the final common pathway for aging and injuries of the joint, but also as an active joint disease. As medical advances lengthen average life expectancy, OA will become a larger public health problem - not only because it is a manifestation of aging but because it usually takes many years to reach clinical relevance. OA is already one of the ten most disabling diseases in industrialized countries. OA is rare in people under 40 but becomes more common with age – most people over 65 years of age show some radiographic evidence of OA in at least one or more joints. OA is the most frequent cause of physical disability among older adults globally. More than 8 million people in the UK and over 20 million Americans are estimated to have OA (source: http://www.niams.nih.gov/). It is also anticipated that by the year 2030, 20% of adults will have developed OA in Western Europe and North America. OA is not only a common problem among the elderly population, but also it is becoming more widespread among younger people. In the United States, Rheumatoid Arthritis (RA) and OA combined affect as many as 46 million people. This amounted to a healthcare cost of over $128 billion in 2003 (source: www.arthritis.org). This huge financial burden emphasizes the acute need for new and more effective treatments for articular cartilage defects especially since there are no effective disease-modifying drugs or treatments for OA. Existing pharmaceuticals include analgesics, steroids and NSAIDs but these drugs only treat the symptoms of OA by reducing pain and inflammation. Therefore, the need for alternative medicines has helped lay the foundation for a multi-billion dollar and ever expanding nutraceuticals industry.

4. NUTRACEUTICALS FOR OA – TWO DECADES OF RESEARCH

Nutraceuticals have had a major impact on OA research. Various different nutraceuticals have been used in traditional medicines for the treatment of joint conditions such as OA, (RA) and gout. Until the 1990s, scientific studies investigating the potential beneficial effects of nutraceuticals for OA treatment were predominantly industry-funded, poorly designed and of short duration. However, over the past 20 years, an increase in the number of randomized clinical trials and mechanistic studies for potential nutraceuticals has

---

[3] http://www.who.int/healthinfo/statistics/bod_osteoarthritis.pdf
[4] http://whqlibdoc.who.int/bulletin/2003/Vol81-No9/bulletin_2003_81(9)_630.pdf

increased. In fact, a recent review identified 52 randomized clinical trials investigating the effects of nutraceuticals and functional foods in OA that had been published as peer-reviewed journal articles [28]. Nevertheless, the mechanism of action and efficacy of many nutraceuticals has not been fully elucidated, thus providing a major opportunity for research and innovation in this field. Despite this, public interest in the beneficial effects of nutraceuticals is high and many lay publications advocate their use.

Although the exact mechanism of action of some nutraceuticals remains elusive, nutrients are capable of influencing gene expression at various levels by altering DNA synthesis and methylation, as well as mRNA stability [29, 30]. Further, many nutraceutical functional ingredients have been shown to directly act on gene transcription by influencing nuclear reception activation, controlling the half-life of transcription factors, and regulating co-activator activity [31]. Thus, nutraceuticals have the potential to act at a number of levels in the treatment of OA.

Initial studies investigating potentially nutritional supplements as therapies for OA focused on the effects of fatty acids and vitamins, such as vitamin B12 [32]. Since then, many compounds have been studied, both in formal randomized clinical trials as well as *in vitro* laboratory based experiments. Various lipids (avocado/soybean unsaponifiables, i omega 3 polyunsaturated fatty acids (PUFAs), and extracts from the New Zealand green-lipped mussel (*Perna canaliculus*), vitamins (Vitamins C, E and B), minerals (magnesium, copper, selenium, zinc and boron), phytochemicals (curcumin and resveratrol), flavanoids, extracts of plants such as rose-hip (*Rosa canina*), willow bark (*Salix sp.*), ginger, as well as animal products (glucosamine and chondroitin-sulfate) have and continue to be potential candidates for OA therapy.

4.1. Lipids

4.1.1. Avocado/soybean unsaponifiable (ASU) residues

The avocado/soybean unsaponifiable (ASU) residues consist of 1/3 avocado oil and 2/3 soybean unsaponifiables (the oily fractions that do not produce soap after hydrolysis) [33]. This is the most commonly studied lipid mixture, commercially provided as Piascledine (Expanscience, Courbevoie, France). Several double-blind randomized clinical trials have demonstrated a significant reduction in pain following three month administration of 300 mg daily ASUs in patients with OA, reducing NSAID intake. There is a 2-month delayed onset of action, and some residual symptomatic effects associated with ASU administration. Longer-term effects of ASUs have yet to be determined. The observed reduction in pain following ASU administration may be the result of the inhibitory action on various molecules observed *in vitro*. For example, ASUs have been demonstrated to inhibit interleukin (IL)-1β-induced collagenase activity by inhibiting matrix metalloproteinase (MMP)-3, pro-inflammatory cytokines (IL-6, IL-8) and prostaglandin E2 (PGE$_2$), as well as reducing basal aggrecan synthesis [33, 34]. In addition, ASUs stimulate matrix synthesis by activating transforming growth factor (TGF)-β and the MMP-inhibitor, plasminogen activator inhibitor (PAI)-1 [35].

4.1.2. Omega-3 PUFAs

Omega-3 PUFAs such as linoleic acid and eicosapentenoic acid are found in soybean and canola oils, fish oils, flaxseeds and walnuts. A high dietary intake of omega-3 PUFAs is associated with a lower incidence of cardiovascular and inflammatory diseases in modern eastern and pre-industrialized western societies, compared with modern western societies. Although no evidence is currently available from randomized clinical trials to suggest that omega-3 PUFAs are beneficial for the treatment of OA, *in vitro* studies appear to confirm the anti-catabolic and anti-inflammatory properties of omega-3 PUFAs. Omega-3 PUFAs specifically reduce the IL-1β-induced mRNA and protein expression of catabolic factors such as aggrecanase as well as numerous MMPs (MMP-2, -3, -9 and -13), associated with cartilage degeneration [36-38]. Furthermore, while administration of between 10 and 100 μg/ml of omega-3 PUFAs to chondrocytes did not affect spontaneous or IL-1-induced glycosaminoglycan (GAG) synthesis, they did inhibit the IL-1-induced GAG degradation. Finally, omega-3 PUFA administration decreased IL-1-induced mRNA expression of COX-2, 5-LOX, IL-1α and tumor necrosis factor (TNF)-α [36, 37, 39, 40].

4.1.3. Lipid Extract from New Zealand Green-Lipped Mussel (Perna Canaliculus)

The anecdotal observation that coastal New Zealand Maoris who regularly consume Green-Lipped Mussels (GLM) have a lower incidence of OA than inland-dwelling Maoris led to the development in 1974 of a freeze-dried, concentrated powder, marketed as Seatone™ (McFarlane Laboratories, Auckland, New Zealand). Since then, stabilized mussel powder lipid extracts, such as Lyprinol® (Pharmalink International Ltd, Hong Kong), have been developed. These products contain omega-3 PUFAs as well as various vitamins. While there is some evidence for positive clinical improvement in mild to moderate OA following GLM treatment in humans, poor study design and methodological reporting lowers the significance of these studies [28, 41]. Nevertheless, the general finding of randomized clinical trials is that GLM could be a successful adjunctive treatment for OA by alleviating pain with no serious adverse side effects [42]. Some evidence for beneficial effects of GLM extract in the treatment of canine osteoarthritis has also been provided. Administration of GLM extract has been shown to significantly improve arthritic score, joint pain, and joint swelling [43-45]. However, in some cases, a definitive diagnosis of OA was not required for inclusion in the study, and severity of the disease was not always described. Overall, there is little evidence of efficacy of GLM as a therapeutic option for OA. However, the mechanism of action of GLM extract is most likely due to the content of omega-3 PUFA contained within its lipid fraction [46, 47]. Lyprinol® has also been studied in other inflammatory diseases. In mice with experimentally induced Inflammatory Bowel Disease (IBD) Lyprinol® has been found to be potentially useful in ameliorating symptoms of this disease [48]. Thus, the variability in type and dosage of GLM extracts used in studies should be carefully examined in future studies. In particular, the variation in potency of extract preparations due to the use of different commercial products and dosing schedules should be addressed, as these factors could significantly impact the results of both *in vitro* experiments and *in vivo* clinical trials.

4.2. Vitamins and Minerals

Various vitamins have been proposed as nutraceuticals for the treatment of a variety of ailments including OA due to their antioxidant capabilities [49]. The effects of vitamins C, E, B and D on cartilage health have all been evaluated, but no random clinical trials have been conducted using vitamin D. Such a trial is warranted, as several studies have demonstrated a correlation between loss of joint space and low serum vitamin D levels [50, 51].

Vitamin C plays a number of roles in the biosynthesis of cartilage, as well as participating in GAG synthesis. Initial studies conducted during the 1980s in guinea pigs provided conflicting results with high dose vitamin C administration resulting in decreased severity of surgically-induced OA, but increased severity of spontaneously-induced OA [52-54]. A later study ultimately concluded that vitamin C intake should not exceed the current recommended daily allowance [55]. An epidemiological study reported a threefold reduction in risk of OA progression and cartilage loss associated with moderate to high vitamin C intake [56]. However, as vitamin C intake was assessed *via* a food frequency questionnaire, there could be considerable error and bias in these results. *In vitro*, vitamin C supplementation increases protein and proteoglycan synthesis, mRNA expression of type I and type II collagen, as well as aggrecan and α-prolyl 4-hydroxylase, while decreasing lipopolysaccharide (LPS)-induced GAG release in articular chondrocytes [57-60].

There are eight different isoforms of natural vitamin E, four tocopherol isoforms and four tocotrienol isoforms. These natural isoforms are found in edible plants, particularly the oil fraction. Synthetic esterified α-tocopherols are often used commercially, as the estierfication protects it from oxidation. Recent, longer term studies, one lasting six months and the other conducted over a two year period, showed no symptomatic benefit over placebo [61, 62]. In addition, the longest duration study (two years) showed no structure-modifying benefits over placebo [61]. Collectively, these studies do not support the use of vitamin E as a potential nutraceutical for the treatment of OA. *In vitro* studies on the effects of vitamin E on chondrocytes are also not convincing. While administration of vitamin E can increase sulfate incorporation while reducing glucosamine incorporation into chondrocytes [63], vitamin E was not able to affect LPS-induced GAG catabolism [58]. Collectively, there is currently no convincing evidence that vitamin E supplementation has any beneficial effects on OA [64]. There is limited published information regarding the effects of vitamins B, K, and cocktails of vitamins with selenium, as well as minerals. These experiments and trials have produced inconsistent and unconvincing results in humans OA patients [65-68].

4.3. Phytochemicals

Polyphenols are increasingly studied as potential nutraceuticals. It is becoming more and more apparent that the effects of polyphenols (both beneficial and detrimental) are more pronounced *in vitro* than *in vivo* due to the higher concentrations which can be achieved *in vitro* [69]. This is likely due to poor bioavailability and absorption following oral ingestion. Further, interactions between various polyphenols and other food additives requires comprehensive analysis to ensure that the effects of a single compound observed *in vitro* is in fact transferrable to the *in vivo* situation when other compounds are available. Therefore, the use of phytochemicals as therapeutic agents requires rigorous pharmacokinetic and toxicity studies, as well as clinical verification of results obtained *in vitro*. Nevertheless, this is an exciting new area of research, which holds much potential for the treatment of inflammatory-mediated pathologies.

4.3.1. Curcumin

Curcumin is a polyphenol found in the spice turmeric, derived from rhizomes of the plant *Curcuma longa*. Curcumin has potent antioxidant, anti-inflammatory, anti-catabolic and anabolic effects, and has been used as an anti-inflammatory treatment in traditional Chinese and Ayurvedic medicine. We have recently reviewed the biological action of curcumin on cartilage [70]. Curcumin suppresses GAG release in IL-1β-stimulated cartilage explants [71] as well as IL-1β-stimulated expression of MMP-1, -3, -9, and -13 *via* inhibition of the NF-κB pathway in chondrocytes [72, 73]. Collectively, these results indicate that curcumin is a potential nutraceutical for the treatment of OA. However, its safety and efficacy need to be determined *in vitro* before it can progress to the randomized clinical trial stage.

4.3.2. Resveratrol

Resveratrol is a polyphenolic phytoalexin present in plants such as grapes, berries, and peanuts and has been shown to mediate death of a wide variety of cell types [74]. Resveratrol has been reported to possess anti-inflammatory, immunomodulatory, and anti-oxidative capabilities. *In vitro*, resveratrol has been shown to inhibit IL-1β-induced apoptosis in chondrocytes, by inhibition of caspase-3, and downregulation of the NF-κB pathway [75-78]. Furthermore, resveratrol can suppress NF-κB-dependent pro-inflammatory products such as PGE2, leukotriene B (LTB)4, COX-2, MMP-1, MMP-3 and MMP-13. These results support a role for resveratrol in the treatment of OA. However, to date, no randomized clinical trials have been conducted to test the *in vivo* efficacy and safety of resveratrol. A recent study recommends the use of curcumin/resveratrol cocktails as a potential treatment for OA due to their combined effects on anti-inflammatory and anti-apoptotic capabilities *via* inhibition of various components of the NF-κB pathway [77].

4.3.3. Rosehip (Rosa Canina) Powder

Rosehip powder is extracted from the seeds and husks of the fruits of a sub-type of *Rosa canina* and has been used extensively in traditional medicine in tea, taken 3 to 4 times per day. Rosehip powder contains considerable amounts of vitamin C. *In vitro*, rosehip preparations demonstrate anti-inflammatory and anti-oxidative properties, and have been shown to inhibit the expression of iNOS, IL-1α and MMP-9, as well as IL-1β-induced ADAMTS-4, MMP-1, MMP-13, IL-1α and IL-8 in chondrocytes. The likely mechanism of action is *via* the specific galactolipid constituent known as GOPO. Results of randomized clinical trials are inconsistent, with some studies observing an improvement in pain and joint function, and others not [79, 80]. However, there is some evidence that rosehip does reduce pain, although its efficacy and safety require further investigation in large, long-scale randomized clinical trials.

4.4. Glucosamine and Chondroitin-Sulfate

Glucosamine and chondroitin-sulfate are both components of the extracellular matrix of articular cartilage. Both have been used for their medicinal properties for the last four decades, and as a therapeutic agent for OA in Europe and Asia for the last 20 years. During the late 1990s due to the publication of various lay articles promoting their benefits, the popularity of these nutraceuticals increased dramatically [81]. Over the past 20 years, numerous publications have investigated the efficacy and benefit of glucosamine and chondroitin-sulfate in the treatment of OA, by assessing outcomes such as joint space narrowing, functionality and pain. As for studies investigating other potential nutraceuticals, these studies are often criticized for their small sample sizes, short duration of therapy, potential for bias due to sponsorship by the manufacturer, and various other shortcomings [81]. Nevertheless, there is compelling evidence that these substances do possess possible disease-modifying effects. We refer the readers to a critical review article we published in 2005 for further details on glucosamine and chondroitin-sulfate [82].

5. REGULATION OF NUTRACEUTICALS – WHY AND HOW?

There is very little or no regulation of nutraceuticals. The United States Congress, in the Dietary Supplement Health and Education Act (DSHEA), established a framework for regulation of dietary supplements by the FDA [83]. For dietary supplements, the FDA regulates labeling to limit health claims, but is not empowered to insist on rigorous studies establishing safety before marketing (as would be required for drugs or food additives). This creates a substantial potential risk to the health of the public, and serious adverse effects have been reported from some dietary supplements that are currently being marketed. Zeisel [83] has recommended that regulations should be put in place to require that these nutraceuticals are judged as safe before they are marketed.

6. PROBLEMS WITH THE CURRENT REGULATORY FRAMEWORK FOR NUTRACEUTICALS

The current regulatory framework for nutraceuticals is inadequate. Nutraceutical products in general terms cover health promotion, "optimal nutrition" the concept of enhanced performance, both physically and mentally, and reduction of disease risk factors [84]. A recent review by Gulati and Berry Ottoway [84] has focused on legislation governing botanical-sourced nutraceuticals in the European Union (EU). This review suggests that nutraceuticals derived from botanical extracts present additional problems because of their complex nature and varying composition particularly with respect to purity, quality, safety and overall efficacy [84]. The authors have also provided a comprehensive summary of the issue of "grading of evidence" to substantiate different claims and to establish standards.

6.1. Purity

The issue of nutraceutical purity will be highlighted using chondroitin sulfate as an example. Chondroitin sulfate is a very heterogeneous polysaccharide in terms of relative molecular mass, charge density, chemical properties, biological and pharmacological activities [85]. Chondroitin sulfate is currently recommended by the European League Against Rheumatism (EULAR) as a SYSADOA (symptomatic slow acting drug for osteoarthritis) in Europe for the treatment of knee and hand osteoarthritis based on research evidence and meta-analysis of numerous clinical studies [86]. Recent clinical trials demonstrated its possible structure-modifying effects. Chondroitin sulfate, alone or in combination with glucosamine or other ingredients, is also utilized as a nutraceutical in dietary supplements in Europe and the USA. However, chondroitin sulfate is derived from various animal sources by extraction and purification processes. Consequently, the source material, the manufacturing processes, the presence of contaminants and other factors contribute to the overall biological actions of chondroitin sulfate. Pharmaceutical-grade formulations of chondroitin sulfate have been found to be of a generally high and standardized quality and purity [85, 86]. However, this is not likely to be the case for all the products currently on the market; the quality of chondroitin sulfate produced by several manufacturers is poor. There are no regulations in the EU or the US that govern the origin of the animal ingredients in chondroitin sulfate containing nutraceuticals. Therefore, the poor quality of some chondroitin sulfate nutraceuticals has prompted suggestions that stricter regulations should be introduced to guarantee the quality of these products for human consumption [86]. Furthermore, it has strongly been recommended that pharmaceutical-grade chondroitin sulfate should be used rather than food-grade supplements. This is likely to have huge financial implications and may result in non-compliance by some manufacturers due to the high costs associated with the preparation of pharmaceutical-grade chondroitin sulfate. We can only speculate about how much more complex this issue might be when dealing with herbal extracts and combinational products (*i.e.* mixtures of plant and animal derived nutraceuticals).

6.2. Labeling and Advertising

Manufacturers of nutraceuticals need to communicate the benefits of their products with effective and targeted advertising and with clear labeling. This needs to be done lawfully with adequately substantiated claims. As discussed earlier the regulatory requirements for products intended to cure, treat, prevent, or mitigate a disease differ greatly from continent to continent and from country to country. In the US, food labeling is tightly regulated by the FDA, and advertising is moderated by the Federal Trade Commission. However, the standards and methods used by these different agencies vary significantly [87]. There is similar regulation in EU countries but despite this there is variation across Europe. Global nutraceutical manufacturers must therefore backup their claims regarding the benefits of nutraceuticals with strong underpinning research and keep the evolving regulatory environment in mind. Advertising campaigns and product labeling must not influence their research plans. Only evidence based research will provide the data that is required to satisfy the regulatory agencies' substantiation requirements to ensure that public health is not compromised [88].

7. CONCLUDING REMARKS

In modern developed countries, there is increasing public concern about drugs and their unwanted side effects. Consequently, there is increasing interest in natural remedies, particularly nutraceuticals and alternative medicines. Nutraceuticals with demonstrated therapeutic properties offer a potentially safer and cheaper alternative to conventional drugs. Several nutraceuticals have been shown to have beneficial effects *in vitro* and *in vivo*. However, there are ongoing concerns about efficacy, purity, labeling and exaggerated claims in advertising campaigns. There are still concerns about efficacy and bioavailability of nutraceuticals and their metabolites. Recommendations by Osteoarthritis Research Society International (OARSI) and other organizations about the use of nutraceuticals should incorporate guidelines about the purity and efficacy of nutraceuticals and how they are marketed. Although this does not guarantee that manufacturers and suppliers adhere to these guidelines, it will provide some peace of mind and protection for consumers of nutraceuticals and functional foods in this expanding marketplace. In summary, we continue to advocate greater regulation and regular independent testing of nutraceutical products in order to ensure uniformity, greater reliability and public confidence.

ACKNOWLEDGEMENTS

Contract grant sponsor: Biotechnology and Biological Sciences Research Council (BBSRC);

Contract grant numbers: BBSRC/S/M/2006/13141, BB/G018030/1;

Contract grant sponsor: The Wellcome Trust;

Contract grant number: CVRT VS 0901;

Contract grant sponsor: The Engineering and Physical Sciences Research Council (EPSRC).

REFERENCES

[1]   Kalra EK. Nutraceutical--definition and introduction. AAPS PharmSci 2003; 5: E25.
[2]   Boothe DM. Balancing fact and fiction of novel ingredients: definitions, regulations and evaluation. Vet Clin North Am Small Anim Pract 2004; 34: 7-38.
[3]   Pisetsky DS. Rheumatology in 2006: crossroads or crisis? Bull NYU Hosp Jt Dis 2006; 64: 9-11.
[4]   Murphy NG, Zurier RB. Treatment of rheumatoid arthritis. Curr Opin Rheumatol 1991; 3: 441-448.
[5]   Callegari PE, Zurier RB. Botanical lipids: potential role in modulation of immunologic responses and inflammatory reactions. Rheum Dis Clin North Am 1991; 17: 415-425.

[6]   Arun B, Frenkel EP. Topoisomerase I inhibition with topotecan: pharmacologic and clinical issues. Expert Opin Pharmacother 2001; 2: 491-505.

[7]   Boros LG, Nichelatti M, Shoenfeld Y. Fermented wheat germ extract (Avemar) in the treatment of cancer and autoimmune diseases. Ann N Y Acad Sci 2005; 1051: 529-542.

[8]   Cooper R, Morre DJ, Morre DM. Medicinal benefits of green tea: part II. review of anticancer properties. J Altern Complement Med 2005; 11: 639-652.

[9]   DeFeudis FV, Papadopoulos V, Drieu K. Ginkgo biloba extracts and cancer: a research area in its infancy. Fundam Clin Pharmacol 2003; 17: 405-417.

[10]   Ernst E, Schmidt K. Ukrain - a new cancer cure? A systematic review of randomised clinical trials. BMC Cancer 2005; 5: 69.

[11]   Nair SC, Kurumboor SK, Hasegawa JH. Saffron chemoprevention in biology and medicine: a review. Cancer Biother 1995; 10: 257-264.

[12]   Pardee AB, Li YZ, Li CJ. Cancer therapy with beta-lapachone. Curr Cancer Drug Targets 2002; 2: 227-242.

[13]   DeLuca P, Rothman D, Zurier RB. Marine and botanical lipids as immunomodulatory and therapeutic agents in the treatment of rheumatoid arthritis. Rheum Dis Clin North Am 1995; 21: 759-777.

[14]   Khalsa KP. Frequently asked questions (FAQ). J Herb Pharmacother 2006; 6: 77-87.

[15]   Ahmed S, Wang N, Hafeez BB, Cheruvu VK, Haqqi TM. Punica granatum L. extract inhibits IL-1beta-induced expression of matrix metalloproteinases by inhibiting the activation of MAP kinases and NF-kappaB in human chondrocytes *in vitro*. J Nutr 2005; 135: 2096-2102.

[16]   Shen CL, Hong KJ, Kim SW. Comparative effects of ginger root (Zingiber officinale Rosc.) on the production of inflammatory mediators in normal and osteoarthritic sow chondrocytes. J Med Food 2005; 8: 149-153.

[17]   Park KC, Park EJ, Kim ER, *et al.* Therapeutic effects of PG201, an ethanol extract from herbs, through cartilage protection on collagenase-induced arthritis in rabbits. Biochem Biophys Res Commun 2005; 331: 1469-1477.

[18]   Baker CL, Jr., Ferguson CM. Future treatment of osteoarthritis. Orthopedics 2005; 28: s227-234.

[19]   Liacini A, Sylvester J, Zafarullah M. Triptolide suppresses proinflammatory cytokine-induced matrix metalloproteinase and aggrecanase-1 gene expression in chondrocytes. Biochem Biophys Res Commun 2005; 327: 320-327.

[20]   Frondoza CG, Sohrabi A, Polotsky A, Phan PV, Hungerford DS, Lindmark L. An *in vitro* screening assay for inhibitors of proinflammatory mediators in herbal extracts using human synoviocyte cultures. *In Vitro* Cell Dev Biol Anim 2004; 40: 95-101.

[21]   Schulze-Tanzil G, Hansen C, Shakibaei M. [Effect of a Harpagophytum procumbens DC extract on matrix metalloproteinases in human chondrocytes *in vitro*]. Arzneimittelforschung 2004; 54: 213-220.

[22]   Shen CL, Hong KJ, Kim SW. Effects of ginger (Zingiber officinale Rosc.) on decreasing the production of inflammatory mediators in sow osteoarthrotic cartilage explants. J Med Food 2003; 6: 323-328.

[23]   Sylvester J, Liacini A, Li WQ, Dehnade F, Zafarullah M. Tripterygium wilfordii Hook F extract suppresses proinflammatory cytokine-induced expression of matrix metalloproteinase genes in articular chondrocytes by inhibiting activating protein-1 and nuclear factor-kappaB activities. Mol Pharmacol 2001; 59: 1196-1205.

[24]   Bremner P, Heinrich M. Natural products as targeted modulators of the nuclear factor-kappaB pathway. J Pharm Pharmacol 2002; 54: 453-472.

[25]   Aigner T, Rose J, Martin J, Buckwalter J. Aging theories of primary osteoarthritis: from epidemiology to molecular biology. Rejuvenation Res 2004; 7: 134-145.

[26]   Buckwalter JA, Mankin HJ, Grodzinsky AJ. Articular cartilage and osteoarthritis. Instr Course Lect 2005; 54: 465-480.

[27]   Goldring MB, Goldring SR. Osteoarthritis. J Cell Physiol 2007; 213: 626-634.

[28]   Ameye LG, Chee WS. Osteoarthritis and nutrition. From nutraceuticals to functional foods: a systematic review of the scientific evidence. Arthritis Res Ther 2006; 8: R127.

[29]   Davis CD, Uthus EO. DNA methylation, cancer susceptibility, and nutrient interactions. Exp Biol Med (Maywood) 2004; 229: 988-995.

[30]   Hageman GJ, Stierum RH. Niacin, poly(ADP-ribose) polymerase-1 and genomic stability. Mutat Res 2001; 475: 45-56.

[31]   Shay NF, Banz WJ. Regulation of gene transcription by botanicals: novel regulatory mechanisms. Annu Rev Nutr 2005; 25: 297-315.

[32]   Hallahan JD. Symptomatic relief of osteo-arthritis and osteoporosis with vitamin B12. Am Pract Dig Treat 1952; 3: 27-32.

[33] Henrotin YE, Labasse AH, Jaspar JM *et al.* Effects of three avocado/soybean unsaponifiable mixtures on metalloproteinases, cytokines and prostaglandin E2 production by human articular chondrocytes. Clin Rheumatol 1998; 17: 31-39.

[34] Henrotin YE, Sanchez C, Deberg MA *et al.* Avocado/soybean unsaponifiables increase aggrecan synthesis and reduce catabolic and proinflammatory mediator production by human osteoarthritic chondrocytes. J Rheumatol 2003; 30: 1825-1834.

[35] Boumediene K, Felisaz N, Bogdanowicz P, Galera P, Guillou GB, Pujol JP. Avocado/soya unsaponifiables enhance the expression of transforming growth factor beta1 and beta2 in cultured articular chondrocytes. Arthritis Rheum 1999; 42: 148-156.

[36] Curtis CL, Hughes CE, Flannery CR, Little CB, Harwood JL, Caterson B. n-3 fatty acids specifically modulate catabolic factors involved in articular cartilage degradation. J Biol Chem 2000; 275: 721-724.

[37] Curtis CL, Rees SG, Cramp J, Flannery CR, Hughes CE, Little CB, *et al.* Effects of n-3 fatty acids on cartilage metabolism. Proc Nutr Soc 2002; 61: 381-389.

[38] Harris MA, Hansen RA, Vidsudhiphan P *et al.* Effects of conjugated linoleic acids and docosahexaenoic acid on rat liver and reproductive tissue fatty acids, prostaglandins and matrix metalloproteinase production. Prostaglandins Leukot Essent Fatty Acids 2001; 65: 23-29.

[39] Curtis CL, Rees SG, Little CB *et al.* Pathologic indicators of degradation and inflammation in human osteoarthritic cartilage are abrogated by exposure to n-3 fatty acids. Arthritis Rheum 2002; 46: 1544-1553.

[40] Zainal Z, Longman AJ, Hurst S *et al.* Relative efficacies of omega-3 polyunsaturated fatty acids in reducing expression of key proteins in a model system for studying osteoarthritis. Osteoarthritis Cartilage 2009; 17: 896-905.

[41] Brien S, Prescott P, Coghlan B, Bashir N, Lewith G. Systematic review of the nutritional supplement Perna Canaliculus (green-lipped mussel) in the treatment of osteoarthritis. QJM 2008; 101: 167-179.

[42] Gibson RG, Gibson SL, Conway V, Chappell D. Perna canaliculus in the treatment of arthritis. Practitioner 1980; 224: 955-960.

[43] Hielm-Bjorkman A, Tulamo RM, Salonen H, Raekallio M. Evaluating Complementary Therapies for Canine Osteoarthritis Part I: Green-lipped Mussel (Perna canaliculus). Evid Based Complement Alternat Med 2009; 6: 365-373.

[44] Bui LM, Bierer TL. Influence of green lipped mussels (Perna canaliculus) in alleviating signs of arthritis in dogs. Vet Ther 2003; 4: 397-407.

[45] Bierer TL, Bui LM. Improvement of arthritic signs in dogs fed green-lipped mussel (Perna canaliculus). J Nutr 2002; 132: 1634S-1636S.

[46] Halpern GM. Anti-inflammatory effects of a stabilized lipid extract of Perna canaliculus (Lyprinol). Allerg Immunol (Paris) 2000; 32: 272-278.

[47] Whitehouse MW, Macrides TA, Kalafatis N, Betts WH, Haynes DR, Broadbent J. Anti-inflammatory activity of a lipid fraction (lyprinol) from the NZ green-lipped mussel. Inflammopharmacology 1997; 5: 237-246.

[48] Tenikoff D, Murphy KJ, Le M, Howe PR, Howarth GS. Lyprinol (stabilised lipid extract of New Zealand green-lipped mussel): a potential preventative treatment modality for inflammatory bowel disease. J Gastroenterol 2005; 40: 361-365.

[49] Clark SF. The biochemistry of antioxidants revisited. Nutr Clin Pract 2002; 17: 5-17.

[50] McAlindon TE, Felson DT, Zhang Y *et al.* Relation of dietary intake and serum levels of vitamin D to progression of osteoarthritis of the knee among participants in the Framingham Study. Ann Intern Med 1996; 125: 353-359.

[51] Lane NE, Gore LR, Cummings SR *et al.* Serum vitamin D levels and incident changes of radiographic hip osteoarthritis: a longitudinal study. Study of Osteoporotic Fractures Research Group. Arthritis Rheum 1999; 42: 854-860.

[52] Schwartz ER. The modulation of osteoarthritic development by vitamins C and E. Int J Vitam Nutr Res Suppl 1984; 26: 141-146.

[53] Schwartz ER, Leveille C, Oh WH. Experimentally-induced osteoarthritis in guinea pigs: effect of surgical procedure and dietary intake of vitamin C. Lab Anim Sci 1981; 31: 683-687.

[54] Schwartz ER, Leveille CR, Stevens JW, Oh WH. Proteoglycan structure and metabolism in normal and osteoarthritic cartilage of guinea pigs. Arthritis Rheum 1981; 24: 1528-1539.

[55] Kraus VB, Huebner JL, Stabler T *et al.* Ascorbic acid increases the severity of spontaneous knee osteoarthritis in a guinea pig model. Arthritis Rheum 2004; 50: 1822-1831.

[56] McAlindon TE, Jacques P, Zhang Y *et al.* Do antioxidant micronutrients protect against the development and progression of knee osteoarthritis? Arthritis Rheum 1996; 39: 648-656.

[57]   Clark AG, Rohrbaugh AL, Otterness I, Kraus VB. The effects of ascorbic acid on cartilage metabolism in guinea pig articular cartilage explants. Matrix Biol 2002; 21: 175-184.

[58]   Tiku ML, Gupta S, Deshmukh DR. Aggrecan degradation in chondrocytes is mediated by reactive oxygen species and protected by antioxidants. Free Radic Res 1999; 30: 395-405.

[59]   Sandell LJ, Daniel JC. Effects of ascorbic acid on collagen mRNA levels in short term chondrocyte cultures. Connect Tissue Res 1988; 17: 11-22.

[60]   Schwartz ER, Adamy L. Effect of ascorbic acid on arylsulfatase activities and sulfated proteoglycan metabolism in chondrocyte cultures. J Clin Invest 1977; 60: 96-106.

[61]   Wluka AE, Stuckey S, Brand C, Cicuttini FM. Supplementary vitamin E does not affect the loss of cartilage volume in knee osteoarthritis: a 2 year double blind randomized placebo controlled study. J Rheumatol 2002; 29: 2585-2591.

[62]   Brand C, Snaddon J, Bailey M, Cicuttini F. Vitamin E is ineffective for symptomatic relief of knee osteoarthritis: a six month double blind, randomised, placebo controlled study. Ann Rheum Dis 2001; 60: 946-949.

[63]   Schwartz ER. Effect of vitamins C and E on sulfated proteoglycan metabolism and sulfatase and phosphatase activities in organ cultures of human cartilage. Calcif Tissue Int 1979; 28: 201-208.

[64]   Canter PH, Wider B, Ernst E. The antioxidant vitamins A, C, E and selenium in the treatment of arthritis: a systematic review of randomized clinical trials. Rheumatology (Oxford) 2007; 46: 1223-1233.

[65]   Neogi T, Felson DT, Sarno R, Booth SL. Vitamin K in hand osteoarthritis: results from a randomised clinical trial. Ann Rheum Dis 2008; 67: 1570-1573.

[66]   Flynn MA, Irvin W, Krause G. The effect of folate and cobalamin on osteoarthritic hands. J Am Coll Nutr 1994; 13: 351-356.

[67]   McKenney JM, Proctor JD, Harris S, Chinchili VM. A comparison of the efficacy and toxic effects of sustained- vs immediate-release niacin in hypercholesterolemic patients. JAMA 1994; 271: 672-677.

[68]   Hill J, Bird HA. Failure of selenium-ace to improve osteoarthritis. Br J Rheumatol 1990; 29: 211-213.

[69]   Rahman I, Biswas SK, Kirkham PA. Regulation of inflammation and redox signaling by dietary polyphenols. Biochem Pharmacol 2006; 72: 1439-1452.

[70]   Henrotin Y, Clutterbuck AL, Allaway D *et al.* Biological actions of curcumin on articular chondrocytes. Osteoarthritis Cartilage 2010; 18: 141-9.

[71]   Clutterbuck AL, Mobasheri A, Shakibaei M, Allaway D, Harris P. Interleukin-1beta-induced extracellular matrix degradation and glycosaminoglycan release is inhibited by curcumin in an explant model of cartilage inflammation. Ann N Y Acad Sci 2009; 1171: 428-435.

[72]   [73].   Shakibaei M, Schulze-Tanzil G, John T, Mobasheri A. Curcumin protects human chondrocytes from IL-11beta-induced inhibition of collagen type II and beta1-integrin expression and activation of caspase-3: an immunomorphological study. Ann Anat 2005; 187: 487-497.

[73]   Schulze-Tanzil G, Mobasheri A, Sendzik J, John T, Shakibaei M. Effects of curcumin (diferuloylmethane) on nuclear factor kappaB signaling in interleukin-1beta-stimulated chondrocytes. Ann N Y Acad Sci 2004; 1030: 578-586.

[74]   Shakibaei M, Harikumar KB, Aggarwal BB. Resveratrol addiction: to die or not to die. Mol Nutr Food Res 2009; 53: 115-128.

[75]   Csaki C, Mobasheri A, Shakibaei M. Synergistic chondroprotective effects of curcumin and resveratrol in human articular chondrocytes: inhibition of interleukin-1beta-induced nuclear factor-kappaB-mediated inflammation and apoptosis. Arthritis Res Ther 2009; 11: R165.

[76]   Shakibaei M, Csaki C, Nebrich S, Mobasheri A. Resveratrol suppresses interleukin-1beta-induced inflammatory signaling and apoptosis in human articular chondrocytes: potential for use as a novel nutraceutical for the treatment of osteoarthritis. Biochem Pharmacol 2008; 76: 1426-1439.

[77]   Csaki C, Keshishzadeh N, Fischer K, Shakibaei M. Regulation of inflammation signalling by resveratrol in human chondrocytes *in vitro*. Biochem Pharmacol 2008; 75: 677-687.

[78]   Shakibaei M, John T, Seifarth C, Mobasheri A. Resveratrol inhibits IL-1 beta-induced stimulation of caspase-3 and cleavage of PARP in human articular chondrocytes *in vitro*. Ann N Y Acad Sci 2007; 1095: 554-563.

[79]   Winther K, Apel K, Thamsborg G. A powder made from seeds and shells of a rose-hip subspecies (Rosa canina) reduces symptoms of knee and hip osteoarthritis: a randomized, double-blind, placebo-controlled clinical trial. Scand J Rheumatol 2005; 34: 302-308.

[80]   Rein E, Kharazmi A, Winther K. A herbal remedy, Hyben Vital (stand. powder of a subspecies of Rosa canina fruits), reduces pain and improves general wellbeing in patients with osteoarthritis--a double-blind, placebo-controlled, randomised trial. Phytomedicine 2004; 11: 383-391.

[81]   Vangsness CT, Jr., Spiker W, Erickson J. A review of evidence-based medicine for glucosamine and chondroitin sulfate use in knee osteoarthritis. Arthroscopy 2009; 25: 86-94.

[82]   Goggs R, Vaughan-Thomas A, Clegg PD, Carter SD, Innes JF, Mobasheri A, *et al.* Nutraceutical therapies for degenerative joint diseases: a critical review. Crit Rev Food Sci Nutr 2005; 45: 145-164.

[83]   Zeisel SH. Regulation of "nutraceuticals". Science 1999; 285: 1853-1855.

[84]   Gulati OP, Berry Ottaway P. Legislation relating to nutraceuticals in the European Union with a particular focus on botanical-sourced products. Toxicology 2006; 221: 75-87.

[85]   Volpi N. Analytical aspects of pharmaceutical grade chondroitin sulfates. J Pharm Sci 2007; 96: 3168-3180.

[86]   Volpi N. Quality of different chondroitin sulfate preparations in relation to their therapeutic activity. J Pharm Pharmacol 2009; 61: 1271-1280.

[87]   Heimbach JT. Health-benefit claims for probiotic products. Clin Infect Dis 2008; 46 Suppl 2: S122-124; discussion S144-151.

[88]   Katan MB, de Roos NM. Public health. Toward evidence-based health claims for foods. Science 2003; 299: 206-207.

CHAPTER 11

Recent Advances and Perspectives

K. Bennell[1*], F. Rannou[2] and Y. Henrotin[3]

[1]*Centre for Health, Exercise & Sports Medicine, Department of Physiotherapy, School of Health Sciences, University of Melbourne, Melbourne, VIC, Australia;* [2]*Université Paris Descartes, INSERM, Institut Fédératif de Recherche sur le Handicap (IFR 25), 27 rue du Faubourg Saint-Jacques, 75679 Paris Cedex 14, France and Bone and* [3]*Cartilage Research Unit,University of Liège, Institute of Pathology, Level +5, CHU Sart-Tilman, 4000 Liege, Belgium*

Abstract: The previous chapters have covered a range of non pharmacological therapies for the management of OA. This chapter will briefly outline some areas that are of recent interest in the literature and that warrant further consideration and research attention.

Keywords: Volition, gait, neuromuscular.

1. INCREASING VOLITION

The core of the nonpharmacological management of OA is composed of information, education and exercises (strengthening and aerobic exercises). Despite these modalities being recommended in all guidelines, they are not systematically prescribed by physicians. Further, adherence to exercises, most particularly to home exercises programs is often partial at best. Patients often fail to translate their intention to exercises (motivation) into action (implementation). Moving from motivation to action requires a mental process known as volition. In other words, volition is the mental activity by which intentions are implemented. Recently, the spine section of the French Society of Rheumatology and Belgian Back Society argued that volition might be crucial to the successful rehabilitation of patients with low back pain. It is possible that volition is also the missing link in the management of OA and that to develop implemental intentions could be a therapeutic target [1].

2. OPTIMIZING NEUROMUSCULAR FUNCTION

For nonpharmacologic and non invasive therapy, one of the goals of treatment is to optimize neuromuscular function. For example, neuromuscular function is important to optimize affected joint loading during gait. The neuromuscular training method, based on biomechanical and neuromuscular principles, aims to improve sensorimotor control and to achieve compensatory functional stability. Neuromuscular control (also coalled sensorimotor control) is the ability to produce controlled movement through coordinated muscle activity, and functional stability (also called dynamic stability) is the ability of the joint to remain stable during physical activity. To improve neuromuscular control, exercises are mainly performed in closed kinetic chains in different position (*e.g.* sitting, standing, *etc.*) in order to obtain low, event, evenly distributed articular surface pressure by muscular coactivation. This includes the provocation of postural reactions in the injured leg by using voluntary movements in the other lower extremity, trunk and arms [2]. Neuromuscular control can also be trained by using whole body vibration devices. For this, patients stand on a vibrating plate with adjustable amplitude and frequency. The major assumption is that whole body vibration cause minor stress of the joint affected by OA. Examining women with OA, Trans *et al.* [3]. found that whole body vibration led to increased muscle formation and improved proprioception.

3. GAIT MODIFICATIONS

Since increased dynamic knee joint load during walking is a contributing factor to knee OA progression [4],

*Address correspondence to K. Bennell: Centre for Health, Exercise & Sports Medicine, Department of Physiotherapy, School of Health Sciences, University of Melbourne, Melbourne, VIC, Australia, 3010; Tel: +61 3 8344 4171; Fax: +61 3 8344 4188; E-mail: k.bennell@unimelb.edu.au

interventions that reduce knee load may be disease-modifying. Gait modification, whereby a patient is taught to modify aspects of their walking, is a conservative treatment frequently used in the clinical setting for a range of other conditions that is currently receiving attention for knee OA.

A recent systematic review evaluated the effect of gait modification strategies on the knee adduction moment [5], an indirect indicator of medial knee load [6] with higher values linked to a greater risk of knee osteoarthritis structural progression [4]. The review identified 24 studies involving those with knee OA and healthy individuals, all of which utilised a within-subject design and generally evaluated the immediate effects (within-session) of the gait modification (Table **1**). The results of the systematic review provide limited evidence for the benefits of some gait modifications in reducing medial knee joint load. Modifying gait to increase lateral trunk lean to the affected side during stance, increase toe-out angle, perform a medial knee thrust pattern, or use a cane in the contralateral hand have the potential to reduce the knee adduction moment, and therefore offer the most promise for people with knee OA. In contrast, performance of a Tai-Chi gait and ipsilateral cane use may increase the knee adduction moment.

Recent research has also focused on novel approaches to facilitate gait retraining. A knee brace that provides auditory feedback to the user during gait was shown to effectively change the gait kinematics during walking leading to a reduced rate of loading experienced at initial foot contact [7]. Providing real-time biofeedback of various gait parameters using 3-D gait analysis has also been reported [8, 9]. One study showed that in patients with knee OA, real-time feedback of dynamic knee alignment provided over eight training sessions resulted in significant reductions of 19% in the knee adduction moment [9]. In another study, real-biofeedback of trunk lean angles showed that small (4°), medium (8°), and large (12°) amounts of lateral trunk lean reduced the peak external knee adduction moment by 7%, 21%, and 25%, respectively.

Future research is required to determine whether the gait modifications cause adverse biomechanical effects at other joints, how best to practically teach gait modifications in a clinical setting and to evaluate long-term patient adherence. It also remains unknown whether reductions in the knee adduction moment observed with gait modifications translate into longer-term clinically relevant changes. Randomised controlled trials of several promising gait modifications are required to conclusively determine whether gait modifications can substantially reduce symptoms and the risk of disease progression without significant adverse effects.

Table 1: Gait modification strategies that can influence medial knee load during walking.

- Toe-out angle
- Gait speed
- Trunk lean to the affected side during stance
- Gait aid
- Medial knee thrust
- Step width
- Nordic walking poles
- Tai chi walking pattern

4. Topical Gels

Pain relief can be achieved by using nonsteroidal antiinflammatory drugs and analgesics. However, the oral administration of these drugs is commonly associated with some adverse effects. One alternative is the used of topical gel or cream containing natural anti-inflammatory or analgesic substances. In particular, the symptomatic efficacy of capsain gel and comfrey root ointment have been demonstrated in double-blind, randomized, placebo controlled trials in knee OA [10,11]. Nevertheless, additional randomized placebo or active gels controlled trials are required before concludingon their efficacy.

CONCLUDING REMARKS

Non pharmacological therapies are largely recommended in the most popular guidelines, even some of these therapies lack of supportive evidence. More clinical trials are needed to demonstrate their efficacy and the cost-effectiveness of these approaches. OA is a long-term progressive disease affecting elderly people with some co-morbidity. The risk/benefit ratio of each modality must be well appreciated before its application. Patient-centered active modalities without adverse effects should be preferred to passive modalities. Additional efforts are required to better implement nonpharmacological therapies in the daily practice of health professional.

REFERENCES

[1]   Broonen JP, Marty M, Legout V, Cedraschi C, Henrotin Y. Is volition the missing link in the management of low back pain. Joint Bone Spine 2010; doi:10.1016/j.jbspin.2010.10.09.

[2]   Ageberg E, Link A, Ross EM. Feasibility of neuromuscular training in patients with severe hip and knee OA: the individualized goal-based NEWEX-TJR training program. BMC Musculoskeletal Disorders 2010; 11: 126-133.

[3]   Trans T, Aaboe J, Henricksen M, Christensen R, Bliddal H, Lund H. Effect of whole body vibration exercise on muscle strength and proprioception in females with knee osteoarthritis. Knee 2009; 16(4):256-261.

[4]   Miyazaki T, Wada M, Kawahara H, Sato M, Baba H, Shimada S. Dynamic load at baseline can predict radiographic disease progression in medial compartment knee osteoarthritis. Ann Rheum Dis 2002; 61: 617-622.

[5]   Simic M, Hinman RS, Wrigley TV, Bennell KL, Hunt MA. Gait modification strategies for altering medial knee joint load: A systematic review. Arthritis Care Res 2010 Oct 27. [Epub ahead of print].

[6]   Zhao D, Banks SA, Mitchell KH, D'Lima DD, Colwell CW, Fregly BJ. Correlation between the knee adduction torque and medial contact force for a variety of gait patterns. J Orthop Res 2007; 25: 789-797.

[7]   Riskowski JL, Mikesky AE, Bahamonde RE, Burr DB. Design and validation of a knee brace with feedback to reduce the rate of loading. J Biomech Eng 2009 131(8):084503.

[8]   Hunt MA, Simic M, Hinman RS, Bennell KL, Wrigley TV. Feasibility of a gait retraining strategy for reducing knee joint loading: Increased trunk lean guided by real-time biofeedback. J Biomech 2010. [Epub ahead of print]

[9]   Barrios JA, Crossley KM, Davis IS. Gait retraining to reduce the knee adduction moment through real-time visual feedback of dynamic knee alignment. J Biomech 2010; 4 3(11): 2208-2213.

[10]   Grube B, Grunwald J, Krug L, Staiger C. Efficacy of a comfrey root (symphyti office.radix) extract ointment in the treatment of patients with painful osteoarthritis of the knee: results of a double-blind, randomized, bicenter, placebo-controlled trial. Phytomedicine 2007; 14:2-10.

[11]   Kosuwon W, Sirichatiwapee W, Wisanuyotin T, Jeeravipoolvam P, Laupattarakasem W. Efficacy of symptomatic control of knee osteoarthritis with 0.0125% of capsaicin versus placebo. J Med Assoc Thai 2010; 93(10): 1188-95.

INDEX

www.ingramcontent.com/pod-product-compliance
Lightning Source LLC
Chambersburg PA
CBHW041729210326
41598CB00008B/823

* 9 7 8 1 6 0 8 0 5 5 4 1 8 *